Honey and healing

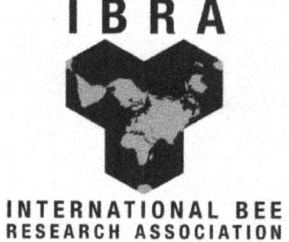
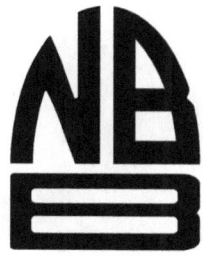

edited by Pamela Munn
& Richard Jones

Honey and healing

Edited by Pamela Munn and Richard Jones

Layout by Design Stage, Cardiff.
Preproduction by D&P Design and Print

©2001 The International Bee Research Association

All rights reserved. No part of this publication may be reproduced, stored or transmitted in any form or by any means, electronically, mechanically, by photocopying, recording, scanning or otherwise without the prior permission of the copyright owners.

ISBN: 978-0-86098-285-2

First edition April 2001. Second Edition December 2017. Jointly published by the International Bee Research Association, 91 Brinsea Road, Congresbury, Bristol, BS49 5JJ, UK and Northern Bee Books, Scout Bottom Farm, Mytholmroyd, Hebden Bridge, HX7 5JS, UK.

Orders: bookshop@ibra.org.uk or
www.northernbeebooks.co.uk

The International Bee Research Association is a Company limited by Guarantee, Registered in England and Wales, Reg. No. 463819, Registered Office: 91 Brinsea Road, Congresbury, Bristol, BS49 5JJ, UK, and is a Registered Charity No. 209222.

http://www.ibra.org.uk/
https://www.facebook.com/IBRAssociation
https://twitter.com/ibra_bee

Foreword to the 2017 reprint.

This book was derived from papers given at the meeting organised by the International Bee Research Association entitled: "Honey and healing: from the hive to the hospital" which was held at the University of Cardiff on 7 October 2000. The programme for the meeting stated: "Man has known the curative properties of honey from the earliest times. We may have forgotten, in latter years, just what medicinal benefits the golden harvest of the hive can bring. Perhaps with bacteria ever more resistant to antibiotics and viruses that seemingly defeat the medical world it is time to look once again to one of nature's own medicines that has a scientifically proven track record".

The book was originally published in 2001, but has been out of print for a number of years. Sadly, Peter Molan, who contributed two chapters, died in 2015. In his obituary published in *Bee World*, his colleague Prof. Rose Cooper wrote: "I met Peter Molan by chance late in 1996 when I was collecting wound swabs from outpatients attending the Wound Healing Research Unit's clinic at the University Hospital of Wales. He was visiting his mother in Cardiff (where he was born and brought up) and had come to the hospital to promote the use of manuka honey in treating wounds. We chatted for about an hour and he offered to send me some samples of honey when he returned to New Zealand. I did my first experiments on the antibacterial activity of honey in 1997, and it marked the start of a wonderful collaboration that changed the course of my professional life".

It is thus fitting that we republish this popular book.

Norman Carreck
IBRA Science Director
October 2017

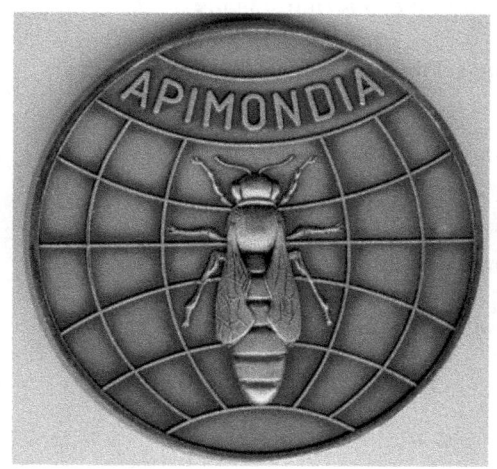

Honey and healing was awarded a bronze medal in the contest for beekeeping books at the 31st International Apicultural Congress (Apimondia) held at Durban, South Africa in October 2001.

Contents

Honey and healing through the ages   1
Richard Jones

Why honey is effective as a medicine: its use in modern medicine   5
Peter Molan

Why honey is effective as a medicine: the scientific explanation of its effects   14
Peter Molan

How does honey heal wounds?   27
Rose Cooper

The role of honey in wound healing and repair   35
Ken Jones

The treatment of burns and other wounds with honey   37
Theo Postmes

Stingless bee honey and the treatment of cataracts   41
Patricia Vit

Appendix: botulism and honey   48
Cliff van Eaton

Important Notes

This publication reports information, but does not constitute medical advice on the usage of honey. Mention of a proprietary product does not constitute an endorsement or a recommendation by IBRA for its use. The views expressed in this publication are not necessarily those of the International Bee Research Association.

Honey and healing through the ages

Richard Jones

Honey is once again becoming accepted as a reputable and effective healing agent — not just amongst the general public but also amongst those that practise conventional medicine. This widespread acceptance and increased curiosity in the therapeutic powers of honey must be due to the increased awareness of the very positive and encouraging results that are being obtained in clinical tests. Particularly the work being done by Dr Peter Molan[10] in New Zealand, and in Cardiff by Dr Rose Cooper and Dr Ken Jones.

It is known from evidence such as bees trapped in amber, that the honey bee has been around for about 50 million years. Mankind, in recognizable form, has been around for less than 2 million years but, from the very beginning, it would not be hard to conclude that honey has figured somewhere in his diet.

Stone Age rock paintings in several different locations show scenes of honey hunting, and these have been dated to 6000 BC or earlier. Thus giving between eight and 10 thousand years of evidence that the human race has recognized honey as a precious product. In southern England there is evidence of honey being stored in earthenware pots around 2500 BC[3].

Honey, therefore, has been seen not only as a welcome food supplement, but also as having significance in religious ceremonies and as a medicine. The oldest written record of its medicinal use is a prescription written on a Samarian clay tablet (c. 2000 BC). This prescription states[8]:

> Grind to a powder river dust and... [here the words are missing] then knead it in water and honey and let plain oil and hot cedar oil be spread over it.

It is thought that this might be a cure for some skin infection or ulcer. There is certainly evidence from about the same period of similar medicines being used to treat eye and ear disorders, e.g. a honey and butter paste was often used after surgery, or to help the healing of stretched or pierced ears. Sometimes, depending on its purpose, the paste was enriched with other ingredients such as barley or herbs.

In Asia, where there are other sources of sweeteners, honey has always been considered as having prime medicinal value. It is mentioned as such in Chinese literature dating from about 2000 BC.

The *Veda*, the sacred books of the people occupying the Indus and Ganges valleys about 1000 BC, record[11]:

> Let one take honey ... to beautify his appearance, develop his brain faculty and strengthen his body.

In Ancient Egypt honey bees and honey were important and are to be seen in many hieroglyphics. The Egyptians have kept bees in hives, similar to those still used in that part of the world today, for over 4000 years and honey was, and is, much used in medicine.

Various papyrus records have been found and transcribed. The *Ebers papyrus* (c. 1550 BC) included 147 prescriptions for the external application of medicines involving honey. One example mixes honey with red ochre, powdered alabaster and a couple of other ingredients to cure 'spotted baldness' — what we would know as alopecia. Similar mixtures were used to: dress wounds, burns, abscesses, sores, and skin conditions resulting from scurvy. Other uses included application of honey after surgery, including circumcision, use as a suppository, and to reduce inflammation and loosen stiff joints.

Honey has been used as a contraceptive: an Ancient Egyptian prescription used powdered crocodile faeces, salt petre and honey. Another prescription substitutes elephant dung. Allegedly, cotton soaked in honey and lemon juice was still being used as a contraceptive in Egypt in the 1990s[4].

Another papyrus, *The Smith papyrus*, gives a remarkable picture of medicine and surgery over 4000 years ago including 48 case studies. One of these describes a gaping eyebrow wound penetrating to the bone. The treatment was as follows[9]:

> Now after you have stitched it, you should bind fresh meat upon it the first day. If you find the stitching of the wound is loose, draw it together and treat it with grease and honey everyday until the patient recovers.

The same papyrus gives many other prescriptions such as the treatment of wounds and ulcers with linen soaked in frankincense and honey, while aniseed, sycamore and frankincense could be used as a gargle for treating mouth ulcers and sores. A most improbable mixture is that of malachite (hydrated copper carbonate) and honey for eye conditions such as conjunctivitis, and an eye makeup for the prevention of eye conditions.

There are, of course, Biblical references to the use of honey and some of these can be dated. In about 1700 BC Jacob told his sons to take '...a little balsam, a little honey...' as a present when they set off to visit their brother Joseph (Genesis 43.11) The Koran too mentions honey when it says that God inspired bees to eat from all fruits to produce liquids of different colours in which there are cures for man[9].

So the remedies of Egypt passed to Ancient Greece and although Hippocrates, sometimes known as the father of modern medicine, does not give it much space, he does extol the virtue of honey saying that it:

> ...cleans sores and ulcers, softens hard ulcers of the lips, heals carbuncles and running sores.

He also refers to 'oxymel' (honey and vinegar) applied topically as a cure for pain and 'hydromel' (honey and water) for thirst, perhaps associated with fever.

It is in Greek literature too that we find a warning about the use of certain honeys. Zenaphon relates how many of his soldiers were overcome by honey that they found near Trebizond in Asia Minor[13]:

> All the soldiers who ate of the honey lost their senses and were seized with vomiting and purging, none of them being able to stand on their legs. Those that ate but little were like men very drunk, and those that ate much like madmen, and some like dying persons.

The good news is that none actually died but they did take 24 hours, and longer, to get over the poisoning. It is thought that this honey had been produced by bees foraging on Rhododendron. There is no doubt that some honeys can be noxious to human beings, but it may also be that the effects of these honeys were somewhat exaggerated by the ancient writers.

Honey was the most useful substance in the Roman pharmacopoeia where it was often prescribed alone or in combination. Pliny wrote that it was good for afflictions of the jaw, the throat, quinsy, complaints of the mouth, pneumonia, pleurisy and snake bites. It is also interesting that he too notes some honeys had a distinctly unpleasant effect if taken internally, but that these same honeys when mixed with aloes made a fine treatment for bruises[13].

A medical writer, Marcellus Empiricus, living in Bordeaux about AD 400 recorded that[2,4]:

> Honey, butter and oil of roses, of each a like quantity, warme helps the pain of ears, dullness of sight and white spots in the eyes.

There is a rich source of information through texts written between 200 BC and AD 400 covering not just that period but the previous 2000 years as well. Then we come to the Dark Ages where there are hardly any records. Dr Crane refers[4] to *The leech book of Bald* of about AD 1000 where honey is again recommended as an eye salve, also for treating sties, dirty wounds, internal wounds, application after amputations and to help the removal of scabs.

Medieval times are generally regarded as a period of medical stagnation due probably to the stifling influence of the church. However, an anonymous surgical treatise from 1446 has recently come to light[7] and this includes a detailed description of ulcer care enumerating seven steps in their treatment Step 4 is called *mundification* — this is the cleansing of the ulcer and gives the following advice:

> *The putrefying flesh must be removed with strong cleansers...if the ulcer is deep and there are crooked veins within it, wash with this:*

Sage leaves	2 handfuls
Wormwood	1/2 handful

Boil these in:

Water	2 pints

Then mix in:

White Gascony wine	2 pints

Strain this mixture and then add:

Alum	2 oz
Honey	1/2 pint

Once cleansed the next step was to encourage the production of granulation tissue. A stiff, protective and adherent dressing was made using the following ingredients:

Rosin	4 oz
Bees wax	4 oz
Tallow	4 oz

Melted together and strained then returned to the heat to add:

Verdigris	2 dr

Stir them for as long as it takes to say 2 creeds as it cools add:

Rose oil	2 oz
Frankincense	2 dr
Mastic	2 dr (This could be propolis, another bee product)

The final step was for easing the pain through an analgesic. The 'recipe' for which was:

Flowering tops of hemp	2 handfuls
Red cabbage leaves	2 handfuls
Avens	1 handful
Herb Robert	1 handful
Clean Madder roots	2 lbs

Crushed into a fine paste, then mixed with:

White wine	4 pints

Strained and clarified using 3 egg whites. To this half a pint of honey is added.

Dosage: 3 spoonfuls every morning and evening.

So we can see similar uses and applications of honey spanning the centuries and crossing the known world. Generally there is very little written until we come to the 17th Century.

In 1623 the Rev. Charles Butler wrote *The feminine monarchie*[1] that has become a seminal treatise on bees. He goes into detail on the production and extraction of honey and describes its medicinal uses:

- For cleansing and disinfecting.
- As a laxative and diuretic.
- A cough medicine.
- An eye balm.
- A highly nourishing restorative.
- An aphrodisiac.
- A preservative.
- A mouthwash for ulcers.
- A gargle for quinsy and sore throats.
- A treatment for snake bites.
- A sobering agent for those that have partaken of mild narcotics.
- A calming agent after stomach upsets.

The first book written in the English language solely on the topic of honey was by John Hill MD in 1759. It has a very remarkable title: *The virtues of honey in preventing many of the worse disorders; particularly the gravel, asthmas, coughs, hoarseness and a tough morning phlegm.*

The book is in the IBRA library and the opening paragraph is particularly apposite to the topic of this publication[5]:

> The slight regard at this time paid to the medicinal virtues of Honey, is an instance of the neglect men shew to common objects, whatever their value: acting in contempt, as it were, of the immediate hand of Providence, which has in general made those things most frequent, which have greatest uses; and for that reason, we seek from the remotest part of the world, medicines of harsh and violent operation for our relief in several disorders, under which we should never suffer, if we would use what the bee collects for us at our doors.

It is ironic that also in the library there is a paper that makes the same point of honey being grossly under utilized in conventional medicine. That paper originated in the Medical School of Hammersmith Hospital and was published in the *Journal of the Royal Society of Medicine*. The year — 1989 — exactly 230 years after Hill, himself a medical doctor, published the same plea. It would be encouraging to think that the curative properties of honey will be looked at more seriously by those that influence our conventional medicines in the coming 250 years.

Many hundreds of tonnes of honey are used each year in manufactured commercial pharmaceutical products and many parts of the world put far more reliance on this golden harvest of the industrious bee than we do in Britain.

In the remote areas of Nepal, where modern transport rarely penetrates even today, the beehive is looked upon as a self-replenishing medicine chest. Similarly in Africa, where medicines are unavailable for reasons of cost or remoteness, honey is an important ingredient in the potions of the traditional healers.

In Russia and Eastern Europe, which have perhaps not had the wealth to develop highly specialized drugs and antibiotics, honey is regularly used to treat burns, open wounds and septic infections. Being non-adhesive it has proved to be not only effective but also more comfortable than other dressings. It is suggested that it is effective because:

- It prevents infection because of antibacterial properties.
- It provides a viscous barrier to fluid loss and wound invasion by bacteria thus preventing infection.
- It contains enzymes which may aid healing and promote tissue formation.
- It absorbs pus thereby cleaning the wound.
- It reduces pain, irritation and eliminates offensive smells.

In Switzerland a variety of pressure sores, ulcers, abscesses and fistulas have been successfully healed with honey when the conventional pharmaceutical products have been tried and made little impression[6,12]. The preservative qualities of honey are not overlooked in the modern age and skin grafts have been successfully stored for up to 12 weeks in sterile, undiluted, unprocessed honey[14].

In the past the only source of food for bees was nectar from flowers. Today bees are kept in modern movable-frame hives and may produce totally or partially non-floral honey if, for example, they have been fed on sugar syrup. The honey extracted from such colonies does not differ in colour or major components from floral honey but may have inferior curative powers.

Furthermore, honeys vary according to their plant origins and the conditions under which they are produced. Processing and storing may bring about physical and chemical changes.

Up to this point the word 'honey' has referred to the honey produced by *Apis mellifera*, the major producer of honey that enters the commercial market worldwide. There are other honey-producing bees such as the stingless bees of the tropics. As you will read later, their honey too has been prized through history for its medicinal properties. The Mayan civilization in Central America used such honey in the treatment of eye disorders and it is used today with proven benefits in the treatment of cataracts[15].

It should not be forgotten that honey is not the only product to be found in the beehive with either nutritive and/or medicinal benefits. The others are:

- Pollen
- Royal jelly
- Beeswax
- Propolis
- Venom
- Bee brood

The greatest problem with this subject is to disentangle the folk-lore from the serious research and then to seek out reports arising from that research. It is therefore a unique situation to have access to so many comparatively diverse sources of information under one roof. The International Bee Research Association has this facility. IBRA has abstracts of almost every article published on this topic and in most cases the full paper is available.

RICHARD JONES, Director
International Bee Research Association, 18 North Road, Cardiff, CF10 3DT, United Kingdom

Why honey is effective as a medicine
1. Its use in modern medicine

PETER C MOLAN

INTRODUCTION

The usage of honey as a medicine is referred to in the most ancient written records[1]. Honey was prescribed by the physicians of many ancient races of people for a wide variety of ailments. Its ancient use as a wound dressing has been described by Beck & Smedley[2], Majno[3] and by Forrest[4]. The ancient Egyptians, Assyrians, Chinese, Greeks and Romans all used honey, in combination with other herbs and on its own, to treat wounds and diseases of the gut[5]. The Muslim prophet Mohammed recommended the use of honey for the treatment of diarrhoea[6]. Aristotle (350 BC) wrote of honey being a salve for wounds and sore eyes[7]. In ancient times honey from Attica had a special reputation as a curative substance for eye disorders[2]. Dioscorides (c. 50 AD) wrote of honey being 'good for sunburn and spots on the face' and 'for all rotten and hollow ulcers'. He also wrote that 'honey heals inflammation of the throat and tonsils, and cures coughs' and 'mollifies the prepuce so that it can be pulled back over the bared glans penis'.

Honey has continued as a medicine into present day folk-medicine. In India lotus honey is said to be a panacea for eye diseases[8]. The use of honey for coughs and sore throats has also continued into the traditional medicine of modern times[2]. Other examples of current day usage of honey in folk-medicine are: as a traditional therapy for infected leg ulcers in Ghana[9]; for earache in Nigeria[10]; in Mali for the topical treatment of measles, and in the eyes in measles to prevent corneal scarring[11]. Honey also has a traditional folklore usage for the treatment of gastric ulcers[12].

There has been a renaissance in the use of honey as a medicine in more recent times. In outlining the resurgence of its usage in modern professional medicine, Zumla & Lulat in 1989[5] referred to honey as 'a remedy rediscovered', and expressed the opinion, 'the therapeutic potential of uncontaminated, pure honey is grossly underutilized. It is widely available in most communities and although the mechanism of action of several of its properties remains obscure and needs further investigation, the time has now come for conventional medicine to lift the blinds off this 'traditional remedy' and give it its due recognition.' Possibly the increasing interest in the use of alternative therapies is the result of the development of antibiotic resistance in bacteria becoming a major problem[13]; or because people are experiencing the sometimes severe side-effects of many pharmaceuticals[14] which in the currently prevailing ambience of 'chemophobia' may be sufficient to give rise to an aversion to all synthetic drugs[15].

There is a tendency for some practitioners to dismiss out of hand any suggestion that treatment with honey is worthy of consideration as a remedy in modern medicine. An editorial in *Archives of Internal Medicine* assigned honey to the category of 'worthless but harmless substances'[16]. Other medical professionals have clearly shown that they are unaware of the research that has demonstrated the rational explanations for the therapeutic effects of honey[17,18]. Many are not even aware that honey has an antibacterial activity beyond the osmotic effect of its sugar content[18-25], yet there have been numerous microbiological studies that have shown that in many honeys there are other components present with a much more potent antibacterial effect[26].

The ancient physicians who prescribed honey for various ailments would have had no knowledge of the principles involved in its medicinal action, just an empirical knowledge gained from its effective usage. But modern physicians generally require there to be a rational explanation for its medicinal action before a traditional, or 'complementary', medicine is given any consideration. Much has been written on the subject outside the professional medical and scientific literature, but many people, especially medical professionals, treat such reports with scepticism, especially since much of the popular literature claims honey to be almost a panacea. The more convincing professional reports are scattered through a very wide range of journals, and some of the explanations for the medicinal effects of honey are to be found in articles unrelated to honey. Hence this review was undertaken to bring together the evidence that supports the use of honey as a medicine.

The first part of this review will cover the therapeutic effects that have been observed when honey is used as a medicine, and the data from observations, experiments and clinical trials that constitutes the evidence honey is an effective medicine. The second part (the science underlying its effects) will explain the various therapeutic effects of honey.

TREATMENT OF WOUNDS

The medical literature on treating wounds with honey has been reviewed recently in specialist wound-care journals, with a focus on the medical evidence[27] and with a focus on the clinical aspects[28]. Here the focus is on the therapeutic effects observed when honey is used as a wound dressing, which will have their mechanism explained later. In the numerous reports in the medical literature on the use of honey as a wound dressing the types of wounds on which honey has been successfully used are very varied (see box).

Of particular note are the successful uses of honey to treat Fournier's gangrene[36,64,65], a rapidly spreading infection that is usually managed by aggressive surgical removal of infected tissue, and wounds from surgery for cancer of the vulva[54,56–58], which are difficult to treat because they are in a position where it is difficult to prevent infection occurring. But the therapeutic effects of the honey that have been observed are common to all of these different types of wounds.

Rapid healing

In several reports the rapidity of healing seen with honey dressings is noted. One report[66] refers to wounds becoming closed in a spectacular fashion in 90% of cases, sometimes in a few days. Another[40] refers to healing being surprisingly rapid, especially for first and second degree burns. Hejase[65] has also noted the rapid healing changes when honey is applied to Fournier's gangrene. Blomfield[29] is of the opinion that honey promotes healing of ulcers and burns better than any other local application used before. Clinical observations made are that open wounds heal faster[34,56] and are ready faster for closure by stitching[34] when dressed with honey (than when dressed conventionally). It has been noted that dressing wounds with honey makes the wound bed suitable early for skin-grafting[41], and gives prompt 'taking' of the skin grafts[33,35].

These clinical observations are in line with the findings from comparative clinical trials and studies on wounds on experimental animals. In one case a patient with multiple ulcers on both legs had one leg dressed with honey and the other treated conventionally (with fibrinolysin and calcium alginate dressing): the ulcers on the leg treated with honey healed much more rapidly[53]. In another case a patient with a long abdominal wound that had become infected following surgery had one end of the wound dressed with honey and the other end dressed with Debrisan (a modern hydrocolloid wound dressing material): it took 16 days with the Debrisan to reach the stage of regrowth of skin over the healing wound achieved after 8 days with the honey. For treatment of burst abdominal wounds following caesarean delivery, the period of hospitalization required was 2–7 days (mean 4.5) for a group of 15 patients whose wounds were dressed with honey and closed with adhesive tape, compared with 9–18 days (mean 11.5) for the comparative group (19 patients) whose wounds were cleaned with antiseptic and restitched[49].

Stronger evidence is provided from the statistically significant results from randomized controlled clinical trials. A trial comparing honey-impregnated gauze with a commonly used polyurethane film dressing (OpSite) as a cover for partial thickness burns in two groups of 46 patients found faster healing with the honey (means 10.8 vs. 15.3 days)[44]. Similarly, another trial comparing honey-impregnated gauze with amniotic membrane (a well-established material used as a temporary 'skin') as a cover for partial thickness burns in groups of 40 and 24 patients, respectively, found the burns treated with honey healed faster (means 9.4 vs. 17.5 days)[45]. A trial comparing honey with boiled potato-peel dressings (another established material used as a temporary 'skin') as a cover for

Type of wounds treated succesfully with honey	
abrasions[29,30]	a fistula[32]
amputations[30–32]	foot ulcers in lepers[25]
abscesses[33–35]	infected wounds arising from trauma[20,34,36,41,51]
bed sores (pressure sores, decubitus ulcers)[24,29,31,34,36–38]	large septic wounds[52]
burns[29,30,33,36,39–48]	leg ulcers[50,51,53]
burst abdominal wounds following caesarean delivery[49]	malignant ulcers[36]
	sickle cell ulcers[36]
cancrum[36]	skin ulcers[25,29,36,50]
cervical ulcers[23]	surgical wounds[32–34,41,54–62]
chilblains[50]	tropical ulcers[36]
cracked nipples[23]	wounds to the abdominal wall and perineum[54]
cuts[29]	
diabetic foot ulcers[25,33,34] and other diabetic ulcers[33,36,51]	varicose ulcers[34,51,57,63]

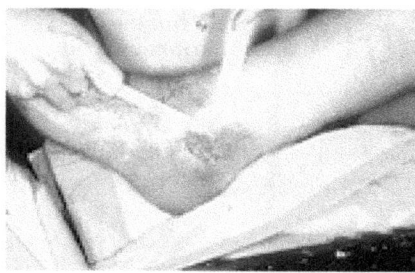

Liquid honey being spread on a skin ulcer.

partial thickness burns in two groups of 50 patients found faster healing with the honey (means 10.4 vs. 16.2 days)[46]. A trial comparing honey with silver sulfadiazine, the most commonly used burn dressing, as a cover for partial thickness burns in two groups of 52 patients also found faster healing with the honey: 87% of those treated with honey healed within 15 days compared with 10% of those treated with silver sulfadiazine[43]. A similar trial with two groups of 25 patients found that satisfactory regrowth of skin over the burn had occurred in 84% of those treated with honey by one week, 100% by three weeks, whereas with silver sulfadiazine it had occurred in only 72% of those treated with silver sulfadiazine by one week and 84% by three weeks[47]. A trial comparing honey with saline dressings in the treatment of pressure ulcers (bed sores) in two groups of 20 patients found faster healing with the honey (means 8.2 vs. 9.9 days)[38].

Controlled trials have also been carried out on the treatment of wounds on animals, with microscopic examination of the wound tissues confirming the directly observed faster rates of healing with honey. In a trial comparing honey with silver sulfadiazine on deep burns on the skin of pigs, complete regrowth of skin over the burns was achieved within 21 days with honey, whereas it took 28–35 days with silver sulfadiazine[67]. A sugar solution was also compared in this trial: this gave the same rate of healing as the honey, but microscopic examination of the tissues showed a better quality of healing with the honey, and cellular evidence of a more advanced state of healing. In a study comparing honey with sugar solution on superficial burns on the skin of rats, healing was seen by microscopic examination of the tissues to be more active and advanced with honey than with the sugar solution[40]. The time taken for complete repair of the wound was significantly less with honey than with no treatment. A study on full-thickness skin wounds on buffalo calves found that honey gave a faster rate of healing than did the antibacterial nitrofurazone and the petroleum jelly control[68]. A study on full-thickness skin wounds on rabbits found that honey gave a faster rate of healing than the untreated control wounds[69].

Other studies on animals have compared honey with saline, a standard moist dressing for wounds. In a study on infected full-thickness skin wounds on buffalo calves, honey gave the fastest rate of healing compared with ampicillin ointment and saline[70]. A study on deep skin wounds on mice found that the regrowth of tissue was significantly greater, and the area of the wound significantly smaller, in those treated with honey compared with those treated with saline[56]. Another study, on rats, found a statistically significant increase in the rate of healing with floral honey compared with saline, but not with honey from sugar-fed bees[71, 72].

Stimulation of the healing process

Some wounds, termed chronic wounds, may go for long periods, sometimes for years, without the healing process taking place. Leg ulcers and diabetic ulcers are common examples of this type of wound. Honey has been found to be effective in starting the healing process in non-healing ulcers[24,31,35,36,41,51,63], some of which had been present for a median time of one year[51], or had been treated for up to two years[36], or had shown no healing over more than five years despite usual measures including skin grafts[53]. Honey has also been used successfully on chronic foot ulcers in lepers and diabetic foot ulcers[25].

Honey has a very low failure rate: in reports of at least 143 chronic wounds treated with honey[24,25,31,33,34,36,38,51,53,57,62] there was only one failure in one report (a Buruli ulcer: treatment with honey was discontinued after 2 weeks because the ulcer was rapidly increasing in size)[36] and six in another (where the quantity of honey applied was very small)[51]. Over all of the other reports covered in a review of the literature[27], with more than 470 cases treated with honey, there were only five cases where successful healing was not achieved: in one report two were attributed to the poor general quality of the patients who were suffering from immunodepression, one was withdrawn from treatment with honey because of a painful reaction to the honey, and one burn remained stationary after a good initial response[41]; in another it was an ulcer complicated by the presence of varicose veins[50].

Clearance of infection

Many of the authors reporting the use of honey as a dressing on infected wounds attribute its effectiveness at least partly to its antibacterial properties[5,9,19,33,36,39,41,43–47,49,53,55–58,62,64,67,70,73]. Honey is reported to be very effective in cleaning up infected wounds[20,33,35,41,54,57,58,60]. Its action is effective even in treating Fournier's gangrene, a form of necrotizing fasciitis which is a rapidly spreading erupting infection that is usually treated by aggressive surgical removal of tissue that has died as a result of the infection, which otherwise would support the growth of bacteria. Honey stops the advance of the infection without the need to remove dead tissue[64,65].

Honey is effective in clearing infection in wounds where other treatments have failed. One report gave the results of treating with honey dressings 47 patients with wounds and ulcers which had been treated for one month to two years with conventional therapy (including antibiotics) with no signs of healing, or the wounds were increasing in size[36]. The wounds were of a wide variety of causes. Microbiological examination of swabs from the wounds showed that the wounds with bacteria present became sterile within one week and the others remained sterile. The outcomes were reported as 'showed remarkable improvement following topical application of honey'. A similar report gave the results of treatment with honey dressings of 40 patients, half of which had been treated with 'the usual topical measures' (another antiseptic) which had failed[41]. The wounds were large and of a wide variety of causes. The number of species of bacteria isolated from the wounds dropped from 48 to 14 after two weeks of treatment. Of the 33 patients treated only with honey dressings, 29 were healed successfully, with good quality healing, in an average time of 5–6 weeks. Another report described honey being used on nine infants with large, open, infected surgical wounds that failed to heal with conventional treatment of at least 14 days of intravenous antibiotic and cleaning the wound with antiseptic[60]. Before treatment with honey the wounds were still open, oozing pus, and bacteria were present. A marked improvement was seen in the appearance of the wounds in all of the infants after five days of treatment with honey. The wounds were closed, clean and sterile in all infants after 21 days of application of honey.

The speed with which wounds dressed with honey become clear of infection is remarkable. Wounds have been reported to become sterile in 3–6 days[52,58], 7 days[36,49,64] or 7–10 days[55]. But, possibly because of differences between honeys in their antibacterial activity, there have been findings of slower clearance of infection: there have been reports of bacteria still present in wounds after 2 weeks[41,53], 3 weeks[47,60,62], and 5 weeks[35].

Dressing infected wounds with honey gives a clean clear base that allows early grafting[41], and gives prompt graft taking[33,35]. By cleaning up the wounds it also allows the wound boundaries to be more clearly defined to facilitate surgical procedures[36,41]. This is of particular advantage in the case of diabetic and malignant ulcers where surgery is often required[36].

Perhaps the most important role for honey in wound care will prove to be in the treatment of wounds infected with antibiotic-resistant bacteria. Honey has been shown to be effective in labora-

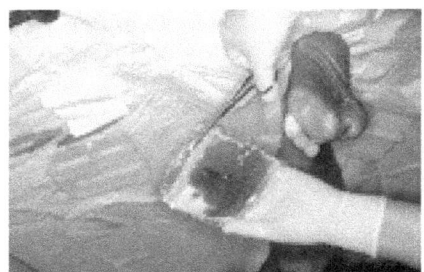

A honey-impregnated dressing pad being prepared for application to a diabetic foot ulcer.

tory testing against MRSA (multi-resistant *Staphylococcus aureus*)[74], and has been found to be effective in clearing up wounds infected with multi-resistant bacteria[35].

Cleansing action on wounds

Several authors have reported the cleansing effect of honey on wounds[29,33,35,41,57,59,62]. The standard procedure for the treatment of wounds is to surgically remove any dead tissue (i.e. debride the wound) which would serve to support the growth of infecting bacteria. Otherwise these would produce toxins which would kill more surrounding tissue. Debridement is a painful procedure that usually requires anaesthesia of some sort. Honey has a debriding effect on wounds so that surgical debridement is unnecessary[36,43,44,46,64,65] or a minimum of surgical debridement is required[58]. Dead tissue separates easily from the wound bed after honey has been applied to a wound[31,36,57]. The dry crust formed on the surface of a wound is also removed by the application of honey[31], and no dry scab forms on burns dressed with honey[47]. It has also been noted that dirt is removed with the bandage when honey is used as a dressing, leaving a clean wound[30].

Infected wounds can be malodorous, especially those infected with anaerobic bacteria. This can be distressing for those who have to treat the wounds, and even more so for the patient, who cannot move away from the smell and who may find it embarrassing. Honey has been reported to give rapid deodorization of offensively smelling wounds[36,43,44,49,54,64,65].

Stimulation of tissue regeneration

When a wound heals, the dead or damaged tissue is replaced by the growth of new connective tissue and a new outer layer of skin (epithelium) spreads over the surface of the wound. The new connective tissue grows in a granular fashion (around newly formed blood vessels), hence is termed granulation. Many have reported that honey promotes the formation of clean healthy granulation tissue[31,33,35,36,47,50,52,55,58,59,62,64] and growth of epithelium over the wound[36,45,47,50,64,65]. Thus it helps skin regenerate, making plastic surgery unnecessary[47,54,58,64,65]. It has also been reported that dressing wounds with honey gives little or no scarring[64].

These clinical observations of stimulation of tissue growth have been corroborated by microscopic examination of wound tissues in studies of the effect of honey on wound healing in animals, where there has been clear evidence seen of stimulation of tissue growth[40,56,67–70]. These studies have also shown a stimulation of the synthesis of collagen, the protein responsible for giving the strength to skin and to scar tissue[68,75]. The formation of other connective tissue components is also stimulated[76], and there is improvement of the strength of collagen[75] and of the healed wounds[69]. The stimulation of the development of new blood vessels in the bed of wounds has also been observed[68,70].

Reduction of inflammation

The inflammation of surrounding tissues that results from infection of a wound, or directly from the damage to tissues caused by burns, is the major cause of the pain and discomfort associated with wounds. The process of inflammation involves blood capillaries opening up and allowing plasma from the blood to flow out into the surrounding tissues. This causes swelling of the tissues (oedema), the pressure giving rise to damage and discomfort in the healing area. It also causes plasma to exude from open wounds, sometimes in large quantities. Honey has been reported to reduce inflammation[40,47,50], oedema[36,46,62,64,65] and exudation[36,40,64,65]. This would account for the soothing effect observed when honey is applied to wounds[21,30,40,44] and the reduction of pain from burns[40,44]. In some cases there is a rapid diminution of local pain[50].

The anti-inflammatory effect of honey has also been observed by microscopic examination of wound tissues in studies of the effect of honey on wound healing in animals, where reduction in the number of white blood cells involved in inflammation could be seen[40,67–72]. The reduction in inflammation seen when honey is applied to wounds must be a direct anti-inflammatory effect, not just a result of removing inflammation-causing bacteria: the anti-inflammatory effects of honey were seen in animal studies where there was no infection involved[40,67–70].

Comfort of honey dressings

Honey generally causes no pain on dressing[54,57] or causes only momentary stinging[30,41,57], is non-irritating[46,57–59], and does not cause allergic reaction[33,36,41,45,49]. In several of the reports of honey being used on wounds the authors have observed that honey has no harmful effects on tissues[33,36,46,49,57]. Over all the reports of honey being used on wounds, with a total of more than 600 cases, there have been no reports of any harmful effects of honey on tissues. Nor have any adverse effects been noted in any of the studies in which honey has been applied to wounds on animals[56,67,70,71,75,76]. These studies have included microscopic examination of the wound tissues[56,67,70,72]. However, there have been two cases where the pain persisted for 15 minutes[51] and in two cases where the pain was such that the application of honey could not be tolerated[41,51].

The pain or discomfort usually associated with changing dressings is minimized when honey dressings are used, which are easy to apply and remove[29,33,35]. There is no difficulty removing dressings[44] because there is no adhesion to cause damage to the exposed regrowing tissues on the surface of wounds[38,47,54,57]. Also there is no bleeding when removing dressings[44]. Any honey left on the surface of the wound is easily removed by simple bathing[20], unlike with many other dressing materials which have to be wiped off or forcefully washed off.

GASTROENTERITIS

The Holy Hadith records the Muslim prophet Mohammed instructing a man afflicted with diarrhoea to take honey[6]. The Roman physician Celsus, (c. 25 AD) used honey as a cure for diarrhoea[77]. Dosage with water and honey is also used by many veterinarians for treatment of diarrhoea in small animals[78], and dosage with an 8% (vol./vol.) solution of honey has been reported to be effective for the treatment of chronic diarrhoea in a horse[78]. Honey has been used at a concentration of 5% (vol./vol.) in place of glucose in a rehydration fluid (solution of electrolytes) in a clinical trial conducted on 169 infants and children admitted into hospital with gastroenteritis[79]. The patients were randomly assigned into two groups, the control group being treated with the standard rehydration therapy (2% wt/vol. glucose in a solution of electrolytes). Testing showed that in each group there were 18 patients with bacterial

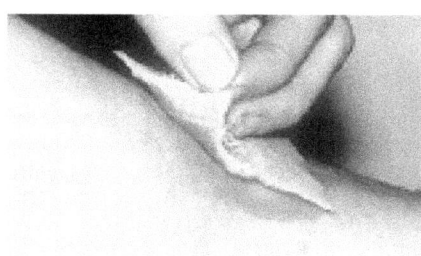

Honey dressings do not adhere to wounds, so can be removed without pain or damage to the tissues.

diarrhoea. The treatment with honey gave a statistically significant reduction in the duration of the diarrhoea (58 h cf. 93 h), and gave no increase in the duration of non-bacterial diarrhoea.

PEPTIC ULCERS AND GASTRITIS

Honey has a traditional folklore usage for the treatment of peptic ulcers[12]. Also there are numerous reports of oral dosage of honey being successfully used in modern times to treat upper gastro-intestinal dyspepsia, including gastritis, duodenitis and ulceration, particularly in Russia and Arabic countries[80–86].

A clinical trial has been reported[84] in which 45 patients with dyspepsia were given no medication other than 30 ml of honey before meals three times daily. After treatment with honey the number of patients passing blood (from peptic ulcers) in their faeces had decreased from 37 to four; the number of patients with dyspepsia had decreased from 41 to eight; the number of patients with gastritis or duodenitis seen on endoscopy had decreased from 24 to 15; the number of patients with a duodenal ulcer seen on endoscopy had decreased from seven to two. The healing effect of honey on gastric ulcers has also been shown in a trial carried out on rats with ulcers caused by aspirin[12]. After 3 days of treatment the control group of 10 rats (given saline) had 15 ulcers whereas the group of 10 rats given honey from sugar-fed bees had eight ulcers, and the group of 10 rats given floral honey had three ulcers: the differences between these numbers were statistically significant. In a similar study[87] the gastric ulcers in the rats were caused by indomethacin, another non-steroidal anti-inflammatory drug (NSAID), which is like aspirin in its action. The healing rate achieved with the honey in this study was 70%, measured as the number of ulcers in the honey-treated group compared with an untreated control group.

Other studies with rats have shown that honey also has a preventative action, protecting the stomach from ulceration by substances which commonly cause peptic ulcers in people: an NSAID (indomethacin)[88], and alcohol[88–91].

OPHTHALMOLOGY

In ancient times honey from Attica had a special reputation as a curative substance for eye disorders[2]. Aristotle wrote in 350 BC in section 627a 3 of *Historia Animalium*[7] that 'White honey.... is good as a salve for sore eyes'. In India lotus honey in more recent times (1945) was said to be a panacea for eye diseases[8]. Honey is also a traditional therapy in Mali for measles, it being put in the eyes to prevent scarring of the cornea which occurs in this infection[11].

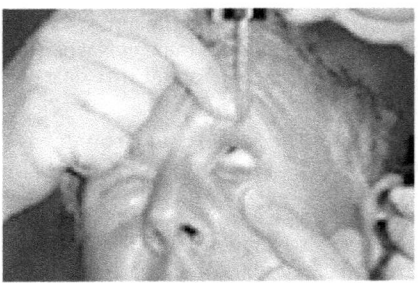

Honey being used as eye drops for conjunctivitis.

Meier has referred to honey being used to treat eyes discharging pus[92]. Sarma, an ophthalmic surgeon at Rangaraya Medical College, India, has been treating bacterial corneal ulcers with honey[93]. The use of honey to treat blepharitis (inflammation of the eye-lids), catarrhal conjunctivitis, and keratitis (inflammation of the cornea) has also been reported[94]: good results in general were obtained, with remission in more than 60% of the cases. Another report has described the use of honey in place of petroleum jelly in a 3% sulfidine eye ointment for the treatment of three cases of keratitis[95]: significant improvement in one case and complete restoration of vision in the other two cases resulted from the treatment with honey, yet there had been no effect when treated with the 3% sulfidine in petroleum jelly. This same paper reported the successful treatment with the honey ointment of 28 patients with various ailments of the cornea, successful in all cases; also the effective treatment with honey of syphilitic keratitis, corneal ulcers, injuries to the cornea, and lime burns of the cornea. It also described a case where a lime burn of the cornea was treated with pure honey, with half-vision being restored in 12 days; and reported that several cases of scrofulous keratitis had responded to treatment with pure honey. Mozherenkov & Prokof'eva have reviewed the use of honey in ophthalmology in Russia[96]. Anti-inflammatory, antibacterial and antifungal actions are seen, the honey being applied to the eye under the lower eyelid. It has been used for chemical and thermal burns to the eye, conjunctivitis, and infections of the cornea, being applied undiluted or as a 20–50% solution in water.

The results have been reported of treating 102 patients with a variety of ophthalmological disorders not responding to conventional treatment, such as keratitis, conjunctivitis and blepharitis[97]. The honey was applied under the lower eyelid as an eye ointment would be applied. Improvement was seen in 85% of the cases, with no deterioration seen in any of the other 15%. There was reported a transient stinging sensation and redness of the eye soon after putting honey in the eye, but never enough to stop the treatment in the 102 cases in the trial. A similar reaction was reported by one of the other authors describing the use of honey in ophthalmology[95].

ACKNOWLEDGEMENTS

The assistance of Niaz Al Somai, Anna Blättler, David Foreman, Paola Galimberti and Jacek Krzyzosiak in translating papers is gratefully acknowledged.

REFERENCES

1. RANSOME, H M (1937) *The sacred bee in ancient times and folklore.* George Allen and Unwin; London, UK; 308 pp.
2. BECK, B F; SMEDLEY, D (1944) *Honey and your health.* McBride; New York, USA (2nd edition).
3. MAJNO, G (1975) *The healing hand. Man and wound in the ancient world.* Harvard University Press; Cambridge, Massachusetts, USA; 571 pp.
4. FORREST, R D (1982) Early history of wound treatment. *Journal of the Royal Society of Medicine* 75: 198–205.
5. ZUMLA, A; LULAT, A (1989) Honey — a remedy rediscovered. *Journal of the Royal Society of Medicine* 82: 384–385.
6. AL-BUKHARI, M ((c. 740 AD) 1976) *Sahih Al-Bukhari.* Kazi Publications; Chicago, USA (3rd rev. edition).
7. ARISTOTLE (350 BC) *Volume IV. Historia animalium.* In Smith, J A; Ross, W D (eds) *The works of Aristotle.* Oxford University; Oxford, UK (translated by D'A W Thompson, 1910).
8. FOTIDAR, M R; FOTIDAR, S N (1945) 'Lotus' honey. *Indian Bee Journal* 7: 102.
9. ANKRA-BADU, G A (1992) Sickle cell leg ulcers in Ghana. *East African Medical Journal* 69(7): 366–369.
10. OBI, C L; UGOJI, E O; EDUN, S A; LAWAL, S F; ANYIWO, C E (1994) The antibacterial effect of honey on diarrhoea causing bacterial agents isolated in Lagos, Nigeria. *African Journal of Medical Sciences* 23: 257–260.
11. IMPERATO, P J; TRAORÉ (1969) Traditional beliefs about measles and its treatment among the Bambara of Mali. *Tropical and Geographical Medicine* 21: 62–67.
12. KANDIL, A; EL-BANBY, M; ABDEL-WAHED, K; ABDEL-GAWWAD, M; FAYEZ M (1987) Curative properties of true floral and false nonfloral honeys on induced gastric ulcer. *Journal of Drug Research (Cairo)* 17(1–2): 103–106.
13. GREENWOOD, D (1995) Sixty years on: antimicrobial drug resistance comes of age. *Lancet* 346 (Supplement 1): s1.
14. THOMPSON, W A R (1976) Herbs that heal. *Journal of the Royal College of General Practitioners* 26: 365–370.
15. KAUFFMAN, G B (1991) Chemophobia. *Chemistry in Britain* June: 512–516.
16. SOFFER, A (1976) Chihuahuas and laetrile, chelation therapy, and honey from Boulder, Colo. *Archives of Internal Medicine* 136: 865–866.
17. SOUTH AFRICAN MEDICAL JOURNAL (1974) Honey: sweet and dangerous or panacea? *South African Medical Journal* 56: 2300.
18. CONDON, R E (1993) Curious interaction of bugs and bees. *Surgery* 113(2): 234–235.
19. BOSE, B (1982) Honey or sugar in treatment of infected wounds? *Lancet* i (April 24): 963.
20. GREEN, A E (1988) Wound healing properties of honey. *British Journal of Surgery* 75(12): 1278.
21. KEAST-BUTLER, J (1980) Honey for necrotic malignant breast ulcers. *Lancet* ii (October 11): 809.
22. MOSSEL, D A A (1980) Honey for necrotic breast ulcers. *Lancet* ii (November 15): 1091.
23. SEYMOUR, F I; WEST, K S (1951) Honey — its role in medicine. *Medical Times* 79: 104–107.
24. SOMERFIELD, S D (1991) Honey and healing. *Journal of the Royal Society of Medicine* 84(3): 179.
25. TOVEY, F I (1991) Honey and healing. *Journal of the Royal Society of Medicine* 84(7): 447.
26. MOLAN, P C (1992) The antibacterial activity of honey. 1. The nature of the antibacterial activity. *Bee World* 73(1): 5–28.
27. MOLAN, P C (1998) A brief review of the clinical literature on the use of honey as a wound dressing. *Primary Intention* (in press).
28. MOLAN, P C (1998) The role of honey in wound care. *Journal of Wound Care* (in press).
29. BLOMFIELD, R (1973) Honey for decubitus ulcers. *Journal of the American Medical Association* 224(6): 905.
30. ZAIß (1934) Der Honig in äußerlicher Anwendung. *Münchener Medizinische Wochenschrift* Nr. 49: 1891–1893.
31. HUTTON, D J (1966) Treatment of pressure sores. *Nursing Times* 62(46): 1533–1534.
32. LÜCKE, H (1935) Wundbehandlung mit Honig und Lebertran. *Deutsche Medizinische Wochenschrift* 61(41): 1638–1640.
33. FAROUK, A; HASSAN, T; KASHIF, H; KHALID, S A; MUTAWALI, I; WADI, M (1988) Studies on Sudanese bee honey: laboratory and clinical evaluation. *International Journal of Crude Drug Research* 26(3): 161–168.
34. HAMDY, M H; EL-BANBY, M A; KHAKIFA, K I; GAD, E M; HASSANEIN, E M (1989) The antimicrobial effect of honey in the management of septic wounds. In International Bee Research Association *Fourth International Conference on Apiculture in Tropical Climates; 1988; Cairo.* International Bee Research Association; London, UK; pp 61–67.
35. WADI, M; AL-AMIN, H; FAROUQ, A; KASHE, F H; KHALED, S A (1987) Sudanese bee honey in the treatment of suppurating wounds. *Arab Medico* 3: 16–18.
36. EFEM, S E E (1988) Clinical observations on the wound healing properties of honey. *British Journal of Surgery* 75: 679–681.
37. DANY-MAZEAU, M P G (1992) Honig auf die Wunde. *Krankenpflege* 46(1): 6–10.
38. WEHEIDA, S M; NAGUBIB, H H; EL-BANNA, H M; MARZOUK, S (1991) Comparing the effects of two dressing techniques on healing of low grade pressure ulcers. *Journal of the Medical Research Institute, Alexandria University* 12(2): 259–278.
39. ADESUNKANMI, K; OYELAMI, O A (1994) The pattern and outcome of burn injuries at Wesley Guild Hospital, Ilesha, Nigeria: a review of 156 cases. *Journal of Tropical Medicine and Hygiene* 97(2): 108–112.

40. BURLANDO, F (1978) Sull'azione terapeutica del miele nelle ustioni. *Minerva Dermatologica* 113: 699–706.
41. NDAYISABA, G; BAZIRA, L; HABONIMANA, E; MUTEGANYA, D (1993) Clinical and bacteriological results in wounds treated with honey. *Journal of Orthopaedic Surgery* 7(2): 202–204.
42. PHILLIPS, C E (1933) Honey for burns. *Gleanings in Bee Culture* 61: 284.
43. SUBRAHMANYAM, M (1991) Topical application of honey in treatment of burns. *British Journal of Surgery* 78(4): 497–498.
44. SUBRAHMANYAM, M (1993) Honey impregnated gauze versus polyurethane film (OpSite(r)) in the treatment of burns — a prospective randomised study. *British Journal of Plastic Surgery* 46(4): 322–3.
45. SUBRAHMANYAM, M (1994) Honey-impregnated gauze versus amniotic membrane in the treatment of burns. *Burns* 20(4): 331–333.
46. SUBRAHMANYAM, M (1996) Honey dressing versus boiled potato peel in the treatment of burns: a prospective randomized study. *Burns* 22(6): 491–493.
47. SUBRAHMANYAM, M (1998) A prospective randomised clinical and histological study of superficial burn wound healing with honey and silver sulfadiazine. *Burns* 24(2): 157–161.
48. VOIGTLÄNDER, H (1936) Umschau und Ausschau aus anderen Bienenzeifungen. *Rheinische Bienenzeitung* 88: 305–308.
49. PHUAPRADIT, W; SAROPALA, N (1992) Topical application of honey in treatment of abdominal wound disruption. *Australian and New Zealand Journal of Obstetrics and Gynaecology* 32(4): 381–4.
50. YANG, K L (1944) The use of honey in the treatment of chilblains, nonspecific ulcers, and small wounds. *Chinese Medical Journal* 62: 55–60.
51. WOOD, B; RADEMAKER, M; MOLAN, P C (1997) Manuka honey, a low cost leg ulcer dressing. *New Zealand Medical Journal* 110: 107.
52. BRANIKI, F J (1981) Surgery in Western Kenya. *Annals of the Royal College of Surgeons of England* 63: 348–352.
53. HARRIS, S (1994) Honey for the treatment of superficial wounds: a case report and review. *Primary Intention* 2(4): 18–23.
54. McINERNEY, R J F (1990) Honey — a remedy rediscovered. *Journal of the Royal Society of Medicine* 83: 127.
55. ARMON, P J (1980) The use of honey in the treatment of infected wounds. *Tropical Doctor* 10: 91.
56. BERGMAN, A; YANAI, J; WEISS, J; BELL, D; DAVID, M P (1983) Acceleration of wound healing by topical application of honey. An animal model. *American Journal of Surgery* 145: 374–376.
57. BULMAN, M W (1955) Honey as a surgical dressing. *Middlesex Hospital Journal* 55: 188–189.
58. CAVANAGH, D; BEAZLEY, J; OSTAPOWICZ, F (1970) Radical operation for carcinoma of the vulva. A new approach to wound healing. *Journal of Obstetrics and Gynaecology of the British Commonwealth* 77(11): 1037–1040.
59. WEBER, H (1937) Honig zur Behandlung vereiteter Wunden. *Therapie der Gegenwart* 78: 547.
60. VARDI, A; BARZILAY, Z; LINDER, N; COHEN, H A; PARET, G; BARZILAI, A (1998) Local application of honey for treatment of neonatal postoperative wound infection. *Acta Paediatrica* 87(4): 429–432.
61. DANY-MAZEAU, M; PAUTARD, G (1991) L'utilisation du miel dans le processus de cicatrisation. De la ruche à l'hôpital. *Krankenpflege Soins Infirmiers* 84(3): 63–69.
62. DUMRONGLERT, E (1983) A follow-up study of chronic wound healing dressing with pure natural honey. *Journal of the National Research Council of Thailand* 15(2): 39–66.
63. BLOOMFIELD, E (1976) Old remedies. *Journal of the Royal College of General Practitioners* 26: 576.
64. EFEM, S E E (1993) Recent advances in the management of Fournier's gangrene: preliminary observations. *Surgery* 113(2): 200–204.
65. HEJASE, M J; E. S J; BIHRLE, R; COOGAN, C L (1996) Genital Fournier's gangrene: experience with 38 patients. *Urology* 47(5): 734–739.
66. DESCOTTES, B (1990) De la ruche a l'hospital ou l'utilisation du miel dans l'unité de soins. *L'Abeille de France et l'Apiculture* (754): 459–460.
67. POSTMES, T J; BOSCH, M M C; DUTRIEUX, R; VAN BAARE, J; HOEKSTRA M J (1997) Speeding up the healing of burns with honey. An experimental study with histological assessment of wound biopsies. *In* Mizrahi, A; Lensky, Y (eds) *Bee products: properties, applications and apitherapy*. Plenum Press; New York, USA; pp 27–37.
68. KUMAR, A; SHARMA, V K; SINGH, H P; PRAKASH, P; SINGH, S P (1993) Efficacy of some indigenous drugs in tissue repair in buffaloes. *Indian Veterinary Journal* 70(1): 42–44.
69. ORYAN, A; ZAKER, S R (1998) Effects of topical application of honey on cutaneous wound healing in rabbits. *Journal of Veterinary Medicine Series A* 45(3): 181–8.
70. GUPTA, S K; SINGH, H; VARSHNEY, A C; PRAKASH, P (1992) Therapeutic efficacy of honey in infected wounds in buffaloes. *Indian Journal of Animal Sciences* 62(6): 521–523.
71. KANDIL, A; EL-BANBY, M; ABDEL-WAHED, K; ABOU-SEHLY, G; EZZAT, N (1987) Healing effect of true floral and false nonfloral honey on medical wounds. *Journal of Drug Research (Cairo)* 17(1–2): 71–75.
72. EL-BANBY, M; KANDIL, A; ABOU-SEHLY, G; EL-SHERIF, M E; ABDELWAHED, K (1989) Healing effect of floral honey and honey from sugar-fed bees on surgical wounds (animal model). *In* International Bee Research Association *Fourth international conference on apiculture in tropical climates; 1988; Cairo*. International Bee Research Association; London, UK; pp 46–49.
73. POSTMES, T; BOGAARD, A E VAN DEN; HAZEN, M (1993) Honey for wounds, ulcers, and skin graft preservation. *Lancet* 341(8847): 756–757.
74. MOLAN, P; BRETT, M (1989) Honey has potential as a dressing for wounds infected with MRSA. *The second Australian Wound Management Association conference; 1998 March 18–21, Brisbane, Australia*.
75. SUGUNA, L; CHANDRAKASAN, G; THOMAS JOSEPH, K (1992) Influence of honey on collagen metabolism during wound healing in rats. *Journal of Clinical Biochemistry and Nutrition* 13: 7–12.
76. SUGUNA, L; CHANDRAKASAN, G; RAMAMOORTHY, U; THOMAS JOSEPH, K (1993) Influence of honey on biochemical and biophysical parameters of wounds in rats. *Journal of Clinical Biochemistry and Nutrition* 14: 91–9.
77. CELSUS (c. 25 AD) 1935) *De medicina*. Heinemann; London, UK.
78. LINNETT, P (1996) Honey for equine diarrhoea. *Control and Therapy* 1996: 906.
79. HAFFEJEE, I E; MOOSA, A (1985) Honey in the treatment of infantile gastroenteritis. *British Medical Journal* 290: 1866–1867.

80. AMERICAN BEE JOURNAL (1982) Hospitals using honey as a fast new antibiotic. *American Bee Journal* 122(4): 247.

81. KHOTKINA, M L (1955) Honey as part of therapy for patients with stomach ulcers. *Collection of papers from the Irkutsk State Medical Institute*; pp 252–262.

82. MEN'SHIKOV, F K; FEIDMAN, S I (1949) Curing stomach ulcers with honey. *Sovetskaya Meditsina* 10: 13–14.

83. MLADENOV, S (1974) Present problems of apitherapy. *International symposium on apitherapy; 1974; Madrid, Spain.* Apimondia Publishing House; Bucharest, Romania.

84. SALEM, S N (1981) Honey regimen in gastrointestinal disorders. *Bulletin of Islamic Medicine* 1: 358–62.

85. SLOBODIANIUK, A A; SLOBODIANIUK, M S (1969) *Complex treatment of gastritis patients with high stomach secretion in combination with (and without) a 15–20% solution of honey.* Ufa: Bashkir. Khniz. izd-vo.

86. YOIRISH, N (1977) *Curative properties of honey & bee venom.* New Glide Publications; San Francisco, USA; 198 pp.

87. ALI, A T M (1995) Natural honey accelerates healing of indomethacin-induced antral ulcers in rats. *Saudi Medical Journal* 16(2): 161–166.

88. ALI, A T M M; AL-HUMAYYD, M S; MADAN, B R (1990) Natural honey prevents indomethacin- and ethanol-induced gastric lesions in rats. *Saudi Medical Journal* 11(4): 275–279.

89. ALI, A T M M (1995) Natural honey exerts its protective effects against ethanol-induced gastric lesions in rats by preventing depletion of glandular nonprotein sulfhydryls. *Tropical Gastroenterology* 16(1): 18–26.

90. ALI, A T M M (1991) Prevention of ethanol-induced gastric lesions in rats by natural honey, and its possible mechanism of action. *Scandinavian Journal of Gastroenterology* 26: 281–288.

91. AL-SWAYEH, O A; ALI, A T M (1998) Effect of ablation of capsaicinsensitive neurons on gastric protection by honey and sucralfate. *HepatoGastroenterology* 45(19): 297–302.

92. MEIER, K E; FREITAG, G (1955) Über die antibiotischen Eigenschaften von Sacchariden und Bienenhonig. *Zeitschrift für Hygiene und Infektionskrankheiten* 141: 326–332.

93. SARMA, M C (1988) Honey in the treatment of bacterial corneal ulcers. Personal communication cited in Efem, S E E; Udoh, K T; Iwara, C I (1992) The antimicrobial spectrum of honey and its clinical significance. *Infection* 20(4): 227–229.

94. POPESCU, M P; PALOS, E; POPESCU, F (1985) Studiul eficacitatii terapiei biologice complexe cu produse apicole in unele afectiuni oculare localizate palpebral si conjunctival in raport cu modificarile clinico-functionale. *Revista de Chirurgie Oncologie Radiologie ORL Oftalmologie Stomatologie Seria Oftalmologie* 29(1): 53–61.

95. OSAULKO, G K (1953) [Use of honey in treatment of the eye.] *Vestnik Oftal'mologii (Moskow)* 32: 35–36 (in Russian).

96. MOZHERENKOV, V P (1984) [Honey treatment of postherpetic opacities of the cornea.] *Oftal'mologicheski Zhurna* (3): 188 (in Russian).

97. EMARAH, M H (1982) A clinical study of the topical use of bee honey in the treatment of some occular diseases. *Bulletin of Islamic Medicine* 2(5): 422–425.

PETER MOLAN

Honey Research Unit, Department of Biological Sciences, University of Waikato, Hamilton, New Zealand

Why honey is effective as a medicine
2. The scientific explanation of its effects

PETER C MOLAN

THERAPEUTIC PROPERTIES OF HONEY

Antibacterial activity

The large volume of published literature from laboratory studies that has established that honey has significant antibacterial activity has been comprehensively reviewed[92,93]. Since then there have been many other studies reported[5,14,15,24,37,38,40,51,53,55,67,104,110,122,144,145]. But much of the published work establishing the sensitivity of bacteria to honey has unfortunately not taken into account the marked variation in potency of different honeys. However, some studies have used honeys with median levels of activity so that the sensitivity of various species of bacteria to typical honeys could be determined. In one of these studies[150] the non-peroxide antibacterial activity of a typical manuka (*Leptospermum scoparium*) honey was tested against seven major wound-infecting species of bacteria in comparison with a typical honey with activity due to hydrogen peroxide. The MIC (minimum inhibitory concentration) of honey was found to range from 1.8% to 10.8% (v/v), i.e. the honey had sufficient antibacterial potency to still be able to stop bacterial growth if diluted at least nine times, and up to 56 times for *Staphylococcus aureus*, the most common wound pathogen. In another study of the same honeys against 20 isolates of *Pseudomonas* from infected wounds[37], the mean MIC was found to be 6.9% (v/v) (range 5.5% to 8.7%) for the manuka honey and 7.1% (v/v) (range 5.8% to 9.0%) for the other honey. A similar study with a range of clinical isolates of *S. aureus*[38] found the MIC to be between 2% and 3% (v/v) for the manuka honey and 3% and 4% (v/v) for the other honey.

There is also clinical evidence for the antibacterial activity of honey being sufficient to achieve a therapeutic effect. In a clinical trial of honey for the treatment of diarrhoea it was found that administering honey halved the duration of diarrhoea caused by bacterial infection[64]. There are also reports of infected wounds dressed with honey becoming sterile in 3–6 days[25,31], 7 days[49,50,108] or 7–10 days[17], and the advance of infection through tissues halted[50,70]. Also it has been reported that honey provides a protective barrier that prevents wounds from becoming infected[20,49,91,128,129], and thus protects patients in hospital from cross-infection[55]. The clinical significance of the antibacterial activity of honey can be seen in reports of honey being effective on wounds not responding to conventional therapy with antibiotics and antiseptics[47,49,66,74,101,141,143,152] and a wound infected with the antibiotic-resistant MRSA (methicillin-resistant *Staphylococcus aureus*)[48].

The antibacterial activity of honey is very important therapeutically, especially in situations where the body's immune response is insufficient to clear infection. Bacteria often produce protein-digesting enzymes, which can be very destructive to tissues[135] and can destroy the protein growth factors that are produced by the body to stimulate the regeneration of damaged tissues in the healing process[112]. Furthermore, some bacteria produce toxins that kill tissue cells[43]. Additional damage is often caused by bacteria carrying antigens that stimulate a prolonged inflammatory immune response which gives excessive production of free radicals that are very damaging to tissues[61] (as discussed below). Bacteria in wounds can also consume oxygen and thus make the level of oxygen available to the wound tissues drop to a point where tissue growth is impaired[123]. The consequences of bacterial infection, avoided by administering honey to clear infection, are: non-healing of wounds; increase in size of wounds and development of ulcers and abscesses; failure of skin grafts; inflammation, causing swelling and pain.

Because of the large variation in antibacterial activity of honey, not all honey is likely to have the same therapeutic effect. Physicians in past millennia were aware of this, at least from practical experience, and specified particular types of honey be used to treat particular ailments. Dioscorides (c. 50 AD) stated that a pale yellow honey from Attica was the best, being 'good for all rotten and hollow ulcers'[62]. Aristotle (384–322 BC), discussing differences in honeys, referred to pale honey being 'good as a salve for sore eyes and wounds'[16]. There is a similar awareness in present-day folk medicine: the strawberry tree (*Arbutus unedo*) honey of Sardinia is valued for its therapeutic properties[57]; in India, lotus (*Nelumbium sceciosum*) honey is said to be a panacea for eye diseases[59]; honey from the Jirdin valley of Yemen is highly valued in Dubai for its therapeutic properties[1]; and manuka honey in New Zealand has a long-standing reputation for its antiseptic properties.

BOOSTING THE IMMUNE SYSTEM

As well as having a direct antibacterial action, honey may clear infection through stimulating the body's immune system to fight infection. It has been reported that honey stimulates B-lymphocytes and T-lymphocytes in cell culture to multiply, and activates neutrophils[2]. It has also been reported[76] that honey stimulates monocytes in cell culture to release the cytokines TNF-α, IL-1 and IL-6, the cell 'messengers' that activate the many facets of the immune response to infection. In addition to its stimulation of these leucocytes, honey provides a supply of glucose which is essential for the 'respiratory burst' in macrophages that produces hydrogen peroxide, the dominant component of their bacteria-destroying activity[117]. Furthermore it provides substrates for glycolysis, which is the major mechanism for energy production in the macrophages, and thus allows them to function in damaged tissues and exudates where the oxygen supply is often poor[117]. The acidity of honey may also assist in the bacteria-destroying action of macrophages, as an acid pH inside the phagocytotic vacuole is involved in killing ingested bacteria[117].

ANTI-INFLAMMATORY ACTION

The anti-inflammatory properties of honey have been well established. It has been observed clinically that when honey is applied to wounds it visibly reduces inflammation[30,132,154]. It has also been observed to reduce oedema around wounds[46,49,50,131] and exudation from wounds,[30,49,50,70] both of which result from inflammation. Pain is another feature of inflammation, and honey has been observed to be soothing when applied to wounds[30,81,129,154,155]. A histological study of biopsy samples from wounds has also shown that there are fewer of the leucocytes associated with inflammation present in the wound tissues[132]. What is responsible for these observations is a direct anti-inflammatory effect, not a secondary effect resulting from the antibacterial action removing inflammation-causing bacteria: the anti-inflammatory effects of honey have been demonstrated in histological studies of wounds in animals where there was no infection involved[30,52,63,77,105,113]. A direct demonstration of the anti-inflammatory properties of honey, where honey decreased the stiffness of inflamed wrist joints of guinea pigs, has also been reported[35].

The anti-inflammatory action of honey is potentially very important therapeutically, as the consequences of inflammation can be major.

Although inflammation is a vital part of the normal response to infection or injury, when it is excessive or prolonged it can prevent healing or even cause further damage. Some of the 'messengers' produced by the leucocytes involved in inflammation to regulate the activity of surrounding cells are prostaglandins which cause the painful symptoms of inflammation. Others cause blood vessels to dilate and the walls of the capillaries to open up, so plasma flows out to cause swelling in the surrounding tissues. The pressure building up from this restricts the flow of blood through the capillaries[32], thus starving the tissues of the oxygen and nutrients that are vital for the cells to fight infection and multiply to repair damage. The swelling also increases the distance for diffusion from the capillaries to the cells[126]. The opening up of capillaries also causes exudation of serum from wounds and exudation of serum into the gut in gut infections, both of which can lead to malnutrition if they continue for a pronged period. But the most serious consequence of excessive inflammation is the production of reactive oxygen species (free radicals) in the tissues[56]. These arise through a series of reactions that are initiated by the production of superoxide by certain leucocytes that are stimulated to do so as part of the inflammatory process[115]. Free radicals can be extremely damaging as they are very reactive and can break down the lipids, proteins and nucleic acids that are the essential components of the functioning of all cells[36], so their continued production can lead to localized erosion of body tissues. The anti-inflammatory action of honey has been found in a clinical trial to prevent partial-thickness burns from converting to full-thickness burns which would have needed plastic surgery[132], a characteristic of burns, where there is much inflammation.

The free radicals formed in inflammation are also involved in stimulating the activity of the fibroblasts[34], which is the basis of the body's repair process, normally triggered by the inflammation that follows injury. These are the cells which are responsible for producing the connective tissue, including the collagen fibres of scar tissue, and in situations where there is prolonged inflammation their overstimulation can lead to 'proud flesh' and fibrosis, an excessive production of collagen fibres[100]. The reduction in keloids and scarring that is a feature of the dressing of wounds with honey[50,128,130], and the cosmetically good results obtained[47], are probably due to the antiinflammatory action of honey.

Thus, there are significant benefits to be derived from therapeutic use of anti-inflammatory substances. However, the pharmaceutical ones have serious limitations: corticosteroids suppress tissue growth and suppress the immune response[27], and the non-steroidal anti-inflammatory drugs are harmful to cells, especially in the stomach[26]. But honey has an anti-inflammatory action free from adverse side effects (see below).

ANTIOXIDANT ACTIVITY

Honey has been found to have a significant antioxidant content[60], measured as the capacity of honey to scavenge free radicals. The antioxidant activity of honey has also been demonstrated as inhibition of chemiluminescence in a xanthine-xanthine oxidase-luminol system that works via generation of superoxide radicals[12]. This antioxidant activity may be at least partly what is responsible for the anti-inflammatory action of honey, as oxygen free radicals are involved in various aspects of inflammation, such as further recruitment of leucocytes that initiate further inflammation[44,56]. (The application of antioxidants to burns has been shown to reduce inflammation[136].) But even if the antioxidants in honey do not directly suppress the inflammatory process they can be expected, by scavenging free radicals, to reduce the amount of damage that would otherwise have resulted from these.

As well as scavenging free radicals to neutralize them after they have been formed, honey has the potential to exert an antioxidant action by a completely different mechanism, inhibition of the formation of free radicals in the first place. The superoxide that is first formed in inflammation is relatively unreactive, and is converted to hydrogen peroxide which is much less reactive, but from this is generated the extremely reactive peroxide radical[39]. This formation of the oxidant peroxide radical is catalysed by metal ions such as iron and copper, and sequestering of these metal ions in complexes with organic molecules is an important antioxidant defence system[65]. Flavonoids and other polyphenols, common constituents of honey, will do this[42].

STIMULATION OF CELL GROWTH

It has been observed clinically that when honey is used as a wound dressing it gives rapid healing of wounds[20,21,30]. It has been reported by many clinicians that honey promotes the formation of clean healthy granulation tissue (the clusters of fibroblasts around new capillary beds that is the regenerating connective tissue)[17,25,31,46,49,50,55,74,132,143]. It has also been reported that honey hastens epithelialization of the wound (coverage with a new outer layer of skin)[49,50,70,130,132], making skin grafting unnecessary[31,50,70,91,132]. This growth-stimulating property of honey has been confirmed histologically in many studies of wounds in animals[20,30,63,85,113], as has a stimulation of the synthesis of collagen fibres[134] and other connective tissue components[133], and improvement of the strength of collagen[134]. It has also been observed histologically in studies of wounds in animals that honey stimulates the development of new capillary beds[63,85], which is the rate-limiting factor in the formation of granulation tissue[123]. It is likely that it is the stimulation of cell growth by honey that is responsible for the 'kick-starting' of the healing process observed in chronic wounds which have remained non-healing for long periods[22,49,66,127,152].

HARMLESSNESS OF HONEY

The Hippocratic principle of doing no harm to the patient is particularly relevant to the selection of therapeutic agents, as most have untoward side effects. Antibiotics have numerous adverse side effects, and antiseptics are all toxic to some degree to the cells in body tissues and thus slow the healing process[137]. For example, in comparative trials on burns with silver sulfadiazine ointment, an antibacterial agent that is the standard treatment for burns in developed countries, it was found that significantly slower healing rates were achieved with this ointment than with honey[113,128,132]. (Honey also gave a better control of infection than silver sulfadiazine ointment in these trials[128,132].) Honey has no adverse effects other than a stinging sensation experienced by some people when it is applied to open wounds[28,101,152]. A transient stinging sensation and redness of the eye soon after putting honey in the eye, but never enough to stop the treatment, was reported in the 102 cases in a trial of honey for ophthalmological use[54]. Over the thousands of years honey has been used on open wounds and in the eyes it has not gained any reputation for adverse effects, and this is borne out by histological examination of wound tissues that have been treated with honey[20,52,63,113]. In papers describing the application of honey to open wounds it is reported to be soothing[129], to relieve pain[129], be non-irritating[28,31,131], cause no pain on dressing[91], and give no secondary reactions[101]. Although allergy to antibiotics is fairly common, allergy to honey is rare[82]. It may be a reaction to either the pollen or the bee proteins in honey[18,71]. In reports of clinical studies where honey was applied to open wounds of a total of 134 patients it was stated that there were no allergic or adverse reactions[49,55,108,130,141].

Reference has been made to dehydration of tissues if too much honey is applied to an open wound, but it has been stated that the hydration of the tissues is easily restored by saline packs[23,31]. It has also been pointed out that although a piece of flesh removed from the body would dehydrate if exposed to a highly osmotic sugar solution, when blood is circulating in it this replaces from underneath any fluid withdrawn by osmosis[33].

Scientific explanation of honey's effects

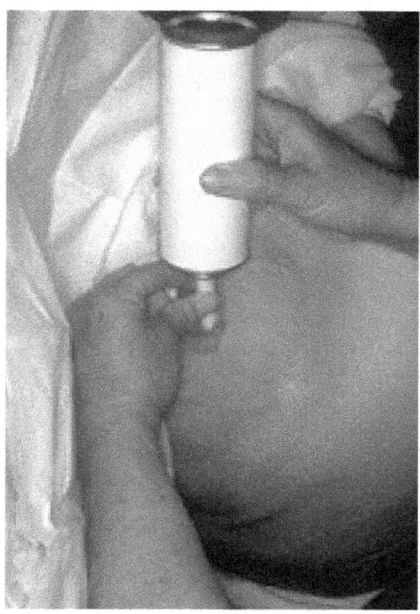

Honey is harmless to tissues so can safely be used to fill deep abscesses. A prototype pressurized delivery system for doing this is illustrated.

There is a hypothetical risk of infection of wounds resulting from the application of honey, as honey sometimes contains viable spores of Clostridia[98]. However, in none of the more than 470 cases in the many reports published on the clinical usage of honey on open wounds was the honey that was used sterilized[94], yet there are no reports of any type of infection resulting from the application of honey to wounds. If spores germinated, any vegetative cells of Clostridia, being obligate anaerobes, would be unlikely to survive in the presence of the hydrogen peroxide that is generated in diluted honey. But any concern about risk of infection can be overcome by the use of honey that has been treated by gamma-irradiation, which kills Clostridial spores in honey[97,111] without loss of any of the antibacterial activity[97].

There is also a risk of blood glucose levels in diabetics being raised by honey. There is also a hypothetical risk of blood glucose levels in diabetics being raised by honey, through glucose being absorbed from honey across the bed of large wounds, but in cases where this has been checked there has been no sign of this happening (J Betts, personal communication). Where honey is taken by mouth by diabetics for treatment of gastro-intestinal infections the risk is greater, but research has shown that honey gives a lower peak of blood glucose than table sugar does because the absorption from the gut is slower[4,78,120].

MECHANISMS OF ACTION OF HONEY IN THERAPEUTIC APPLICATIONS

Action of honey as a wound dressing

The report of G Winter in 1962[151], that wounds heal faster if kept moist than if a scab is allowed to form, was the start of what has become the standard modern approach to wound treatment, the prevention of drying out of a wound. The epithelial cells, which spread across the surface of a healing wound to restore the skin cover, need moist conditions to be able to grow. (When there is a dry scab on the surface of a wound the epithelial cells grow across in the moist area beneath it, and thus leave a pitted scar in the skin.) Also, the fibroblasts, functioning as a rudimentary form of muscle cells, need moist conditions to be able to contract and pull the margins of the wound together. A dressing of honey over a wound provides the moist conditions needed for these processes. The amount of free water in honey is very low, such as would be expected to dry out wound tissues. But the osmotic effect draws fluid out from below the honey dressing, and thus creates a layer of fluid that is a dilute solution of honey in plasma or lymph. A secondary benefit of this fluid layer is that there is no sticking of dressings to the surface of wounds when honey is used[28,91,129,132,147]. As well as giving painless dressing changes, this gives faster healing than with dry dressings because there is not the tearing away of the delicate newly re-grown tissues that adhere to the dressing when dry dressings (or even sometimes the modern moist wound healing dressing materials) are used. Combined with the stimulatory effects on tissue regeneration discussed above, this puts honey in the same category as the latest dressings produced by pharmaceutical technology, a bio-active moist wound dressing material.

One problem with using dressings that create a moist environment is that the moist conditions favour growth of bacteria, and for this reason some of the moister products in use are contra-indicated for use on infected wounds. But honey creates a moist environment in which bacterial growth is prevented by the antibacterial activity of the honey. Furthermore, the antibacterial components of honey, unlike antibiotics, have a high solubility in water and thus can diffuse into the tissues. Honey has also been reported to give rapid deodorisation of offensively smelling wounds[49,50,70,91,108,128,129], whereas malodour is a common feature of the use of pharmaceutical moist dressings on wounds. It is probably more than just the antibacterial action of honey that is involved in removal of malo-

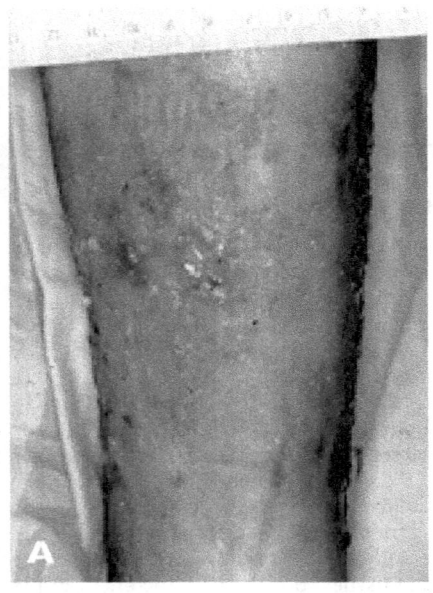
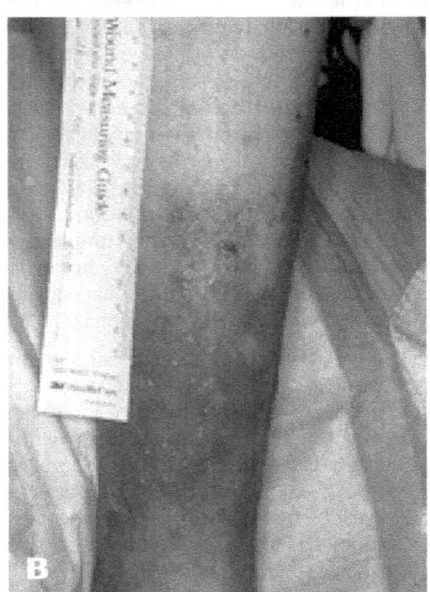

A case of cellulitis (infection of skin tissues) cleared up by one week of dressing with honey. A: before treatment; B: after.

dour: the high glucose levels that the honey provides would be used by the infecting bacteria in preference to amino acids[103] from the serum and dead cells, and thus would give rise to lactic acid instead of ammonia and the amines and sulphur compounds that are the cause of malodour in wounds.

Another advantage of having a moist wound-healing environment is that it allows the protein-digesting enzymes in the wound tissues to work and loosen any scab or pus and dead tissue. The alternative that often is necessary when this autolytic debridement is insufficient to achieve a clean wound bed is to use surgical debridement, as it is important to remove what would otherwise be a good culture medium for bacterial growth[68,126]. A more expensive option is to apply pharmaceutical enzyme preparations, or in some cases maggots that have been especially bred for this purpose. Honey has a very efficient debriding action, such that it is frequently remarked upon in papers reporting on the use of honey in wound treatment[21,28,31,46,49,50,55,70,74,101,128,129,131,143,146]. It has also been noted that dirt is removed with the bandage when honey is used as a dressing, leaving a clean wound[155]. The outflow of lymph caused by the osmotic effect of honey could be expected to help in this clearing of dirt from wounds.

Another beneficial effect that could be expected from the osmotic outflow of lymph caused by honey is increased nutrification of the tissues in healing wounds. Whether caused by trauma or infection, at the site of tissue repair in wounds there are often insufficient functioning blood vessels to supply the cells with the nutrients that they need to grow and multiply. The importance of this is demonstrated by the observation that wounds heal faster if a nutrient mixture is applied to them[80,102,124,142]. The drawing out of lymph would provide a constant flow of nutrients from the functioning blood vessels deeper down. Honey would in addition supply nutrients directly, not just readily metabolisable sugars but also a wide range of amino acids, vitamins and essential minerals[69,149]. The supply of glucose would be of particular importance to the epithelial cells which have to build up an internal store of carbohydrate to provide the energy they need to be able to migrate across the surface of the wound to restore skin cover[123]. The osmotic outflow of lymph induced by honey could also be expected to increase the oxygen supply to the tissues in healing wounds. Because of destruction of the local circulation there are insufficient functioning blood vessels around a wound to supply the cells with oxygen, thus growth of the cells repairing the wound is restricted[73]. Additional oxygenation of wound tissues is also likely to be induced by the acidity of honey, this being one of the two mechanisms proposed[86] to account for the finding that acidification of wounds increases the rate of healing[79,86]. The other mechanism proposed is the conversion of the toxic form of ammonia, NH_3 (produced in wounds by bacterial decomposition of protein), to the non-toxic ionic form, NH_4^+, that is the predominant form in an acidic environment[86]. As an acidulant for wounds, honey has the advantage of having a gentle action because the acidic component of honey, gluconic acid, exists mostly in the form of a neutral lactone that is in a slowly-converting equilibrium with the free acid form.

ACTION OF HONEY IN TREATING DIARRHOEA

The shortening of the duration of diarrhoea by administering honey in a clinical trial was attributed to the antibacterial activity of honey[64], which was in line with the finding that in the patients in this trial who had diarrhoea due to a viral infection there was no shortening of the duration by the honey treatment. (It was of significance that the duration of the viral diarrhoea was not increased by the antibacterial activity of honey, as commonly happens with other antibacterial therapy.) But it has also been suggested that the effectiveness of honey in treating diarrhoea may be due to it effecting repair of the intestinal mucosa (the lining of the intestines) damaged by the infection[88]. This suggested mode of action would be in line with the effect of honey in wounds of stimulating the growth of tissues to repair damage. Both of these modes of action could be involved simultaneously, along with a third possibility, that of the anti-inflammatory action of honey reducing the malfunctioning of the mucosa and the loss of serum from the inflamed tissue.

The routine therapy for diarrhoea is simply re-hydrating the body and restoring electrolytes (salts) lost in the diarrhoea, by administering fluid by mouth or intravenously[64]. The World Health Organisation's recommendation for oral re-hydration is to use an electrolyte solution with glucose added[153]. The active absorption of glucose by the intestinal mucosa is a process that is coupled to the uptake of sodium[64], so the glucose aids in the absorption of electrolytes. It also increases the uptake of water[58]. In the clinical trial where honey replaced glucose in the electrolyte solution it was found that it was just as effective as glucose in re-hydrating the patients[64]. Honey has the added advantage of also containing fructose which has the ability to promote additional water uptake with less sodium uptake[58], avoiding the risk of too much sodium being taken up into the circulation[64]. Fructose also promotes the uptake of potassium whereas glucose causes net loss of potassium[58].

ACTION OF HONEY IN TREATING PEPTIC ULCERS AND GASTRITIS

The discovery that one of the causes of peptic ulcers and gastritis (inflammation of the stomach lining) was infection with the bacterium *Helicobacter pylori*[45] raised the suggestion that the effectiveness of honey in treating these conditions may be due to its antibacterial activity[5,14]. Testing of clinical specimens of *H. pylori* showed that they were sensitive to the antibacterial activity of honey[5,14], but possibly not sufficiently sensitive to account for the therapeutic effect of honey. The concentration of honey needed to stop the growth of the bacteria in one study[14] was 20%. In the other study[5] the bacteria were not inhibited by a 40% concentration of a honey selected to have a median level of antibacterial activity due to hydrogen peroxide, the common antibacterial component of honey. However, with a manuka honey of a median level of activity due to the unidentified antibacterial component of this type of honey, the concentration of honey needed to completely inhibit the growth of the bacteria was 5%[5]. But a clinical trial using manuka honey with a similar level of activity has found that infection of the stomach with *H. pylori* was not cleared after two weeks of treatment with four-times-daily doses of a tablespoon (c. 25 g) of honey[90]. Although it was concluded from this trial that any effectiveness of honey against peptic ulcers and gastritis is not through an effect on *H. pylori*, this is not a reasonable conclusion when the trial was with only six patients treated, and was with a single, arbitrarily chosen dose rate which may have been insufficient and may not have been continued long enough to clear the infection. However, it should also be born in mind that this trial was carried out with a honey to which *H. pylori* is very sensitive, whereas in the many reports of successful treatment of peptic ulcers and gastritis cited in Part 1 of this review it was not manuka honey that was used.

Alternative explanations for how honey has a therapeutic effect on gastritis and peptic ulcers have come from a series of studies conducted by Ali and co-workers, who have investigated the influence of honey on various parameters known to be involved in ulceration in the stomach. There are various causes of peptic ulcers, the major ones being aspirin-type anti-inflammatory drugs, alcohol, and stress, which restricts the blood supply to the gastric mucosa (the stomach lining) and leaves it more susceptible to erosion by the stomach contents[26]. Studies of the action of honey on peptic ulcers in rats have shown that it has a dose-dependent effect protecting the stomach from ulceration being caused by alcohol[6,8,9,10,12] and indomethacin (an aspirin-type anti-inflammatory drug)[10]. At the higher dose rates used, there was around an 80% protection from the ulceration caused by alcohol[6,8], but only if the honey was given 30 minutes beforehand and not if given simultaneously. Only in one case[10], with a very high dose rate, was there any protection if the honey was given simultaneously. But honey gave 100% protection from ulceration caused by indomethacin when given simultaneously. (The difference in time frame of protection may reflect the much slower development of ulcers seen with indomethacin than with alcohol[7,8].) There was no protection from either agent if a sugar mixture simulating honey was used in place of honey[8,10], showing that the protection is due to a component of the honey other than the sugars.

Investigation by Ali et al. of the mechanisms of these protective effects of honey have given an insight into how honey may work in therapy of gastritis and peptic ulcers. Aspirin-type anti-inflammatory drugs, especially in the presence of acid, enter the cells and block their energy-producing metabolism, thus causing the cells to decrease their protective secretions and become permeable to acid[26]. This leads to shedding of the surface cells and development of erosion of the sub-surface, with bleeding and inflammation[26]. Production of prostaglandins, with a protective function, is inhibited by these drugs, but prostaglandins protect only the sub-surface mucosal tissue, repair of the mucosal surface (epithelial cells) being independent of prostaglandins[26]. The action of alcohol is more complex and less well understood, but also involves inflammation[9,10].

The studies on the effects of honey on ulcers have demonstrated that an influence of honey on prostaglandin production is not involved[6,9], but that honey has a stimulatory effect on the sensory nerves in the stomach that respond to capsaicin (the irritant in chilli pepper)[6]. Stimulation of these nerves causes the release of vasodilatory peptides in the stomach which, mediated by production of nitric oxide, increase the blood supply and thus help protect the gastric mucosa from damage[6,11].

A second mechanism of action has also been identified from these studies that involves the antioxidant properties of honey. Honey has been found to protect or augment the level of non-protein sulfhydryls (substances such as glutathione) in gastric tissue subjected to factors inducing ulceration[6,8,9,13], a class of substances that are part of the body's antioxidant defence system[65], and depletion of which is an indication of oxidative damage to tissues[39]. Oxidative damage to tissues through free radical production occurs in reperfusion injury (injury resulting from the restoration of blood flow to tissues that have been deprived of it). The free radicals are formed by the action of the enzyme xanthine oxidase in the tissues, formed during the period of oxygen starvation, producing superoxide from oxygen when it becomes available again[39]. This type of injury is involved in the formation of peptic ulcers[13], and has been found to be decreased in rat stomachs by dosing with honey 30 minutes before restricting then restoring the circulation[13]. Another study showed that the permeability of the blood vessels in the gastric mucosa developing as a consequence of exposure to alcohol, a feature of inflammation, could be reduced in a dose-dependent manner by pretreatment of the stomach with honey[12]. But none of these findings of an antioxidant effect of honey in the stomach rule out the alternative or additional possibility that it is an antiinflammatory component of honey distinct from the antioxidants that is involved. As mentioned above, oxygen free radicals can initiate further inflammation, and inflammation gives rise to oxygen free radicals, thus giving a self-amplifying inflammatory response[56]. The oxidative damage resulting could be decreased by blocking either the oxygen radicals themselves, or by blocking the inflammatory response that would otherwise be giving rise to more oxygen radicals.

Ali et al. have also identified a third mechanism of action of honey in the therapy of peptic ulcers, that of stimulating repair of the damage to the gastric mucosa. Feeding honey to rats with stomach ulcers caused by indomethacin gave 61–70% more healing than in the controls[7]. Observation of the ulcers revealed that the honey caused a decrease in oedema (swelling of the surrounding tissue, a feature of inflammation) and formation of healthy granulation tissue. It is of interest that these observations parallel those made with skin ulcers treated with honey (see above). Ali et al. have proposed[7] that the stimulation of healing of peptic ulcers is by its stimulation of blood supply[6,11], which is one of the mechanisms that is involved in the healing of skin ulcers (see above). The anti-inflammatory action reducing oedema would be involved in this as well (see above), additional to the direct stimulation through the sensory nerves in the stomach. The stimulatory effect of honey on the growth of epithelial cells (see above) could also be expected to help restore the surface cells of the gastric mucosa, which cannot be helped by prostaglandins.

THE ROLE OF HYDROGEN PEROXIDE

Hydrogen peroxide, the principle antibacterial component of honey, is well known as an antibacterial agent, although it has had a chequered history of use as an antiseptic. In its history it has been in then out of favour with the medical profession twice since first coming into use in the late 19th Century. It has been suggested that its ready decomposition in solutions containing traces of catalytic metals such as iron or copper may be the reason why hydrogen peroxide went out of favour as an antiseptic after initially being hailed for its antibacterial and cleansing properties when first introduced[140]. There was an upsurge of interest in its use later when stabilized preparations became available, with good germicidal activity being reported[140], but in more recent times it has again gone out of favour as awareness has developed of the inflammation and damage that are caused to tissues by substances giving rise to oxygen free radicals[65,118,119]. However, the hydrogen peroxide concentration produced in honey activated by dilution is typically around 1 mmol/l[93], about one thousand times less than in the 3% solution that is commonly used as an antiseptic. Also, there is the potential for honey to sequester and inactivate the metal ions which catalyse the formation of oxygen radicals from hydrogen peroxide, and the antioxidant components of honey to mop up any free radicals that may be formed.

Hydrogen peroxide is an effective antimicrobial agent if present at a sufficiently high concentration[116], but at higher concentrations causes cellular and protein damage in tissues by giving rise to oxygen radicals[36,125]. A study of hydrogen peroxide antiseptic has found that there is no bactericidal concentration of hydrogen peroxide that is not toxic to fibroblasts (the cells that repair wounds)[87]. Minimum concentrations reported to be necessary in the culture medium to inhibit bacterial growth range from 0.12 to 5.9 mmol/l[92]. However, it has been reported that a given quantity of hydrogen peroxide is more effective when it is supplied by continuous generation by glucose oxidase than when it is added separately[114], and a study with *Escherichia coli* exposed to a constantly replenished stream of hydrogen peroxide showed that their growth was inhibited by 0.02–0.05 mmol/l hydrogen peroxide, a concentration that was not damaging to fibroblast cells from human skin[75]. A further consideration is that myeloperoxidase, the enzyme that generates bacteria-destroying free radicals from hydrogen peroxide in the phagocytotic vacuoles of the leucocytes[83], is inactivated by hydrogen peroxide levels in excess of 2 mmol/l[3]. Thus, in living tissue where there will be leucocytes active, a better overall antibacterial action may be obtained with low levels of hydrogen peroxide. The action of the enzymes catalase and glutathione peroxidase in tissues will give equilibrium concentrations of hydrogen peroxide that will be lower than the 1 mmol/l found in honey solutions *in vitro*.

But hydrogen peroxide has roles in healing quite separate from any antibacterial action. It has been reported that at levels of 30–100 µmol/l it activates the NF-κB transcription factor in lymphocytes to activate the expression of genes for the immune response[121]. Research on various cell lines in culture is showing that it has a variety of effects in the role of a 'cellular messenger'. A review of the voluminous literature appearing on this topic[29] has pointed out the large amount of evidence for hydrogen peroxide being involved in many cell types in the body as a stimulus for cell multiplication. It acts at various points in the mechanisms of the cells that control the cycle of cell growth and division, most probably by oxidising the proteins involved and thus causing a change in the conformation of the protein molecule. This action has particular relevance in wound healing, where the inflammatory response that is a natural consequence of injury or infection produces hydrogen peroxide, and this serves to stimulate the growth of fibroblasts and epithelial cells to repair the damage[29]. Only where there is excessive inflammation does the hydrogen peroxide rise to levels that instead cause destruction of tissues by killing the cells[29]. Even with these high levels of hydrogen peroxide the cells can be protected by iron-chelating agents which prevent the catalysis by iron of the formation of membrane-damaging free radicals[29]. Without this protection, hydrogen peroxide is toxic to cells at concentrations above 0.1 mmol/l, but only needs to be at levels around one thousandth of this to stimulate cell multiplication[29]. It has been proposed that low concentrations of hydrogen peroxide might be used to stimulate wound healing, rather than the expensive cell growth factors produced by biotechnology for this purpose (the bioactive wound dressings)[29]. But another proposal that hydrogen peroxide could be applied to promote the wound healing process has pointed out that this is feasible only if the concentration could be carefully controlled[34]. It has also been proposed that honey be used in place of recombinant growth factors to provide hydrogen peroxide to stimulate the healing of burns[112]. The application of creams containing hydrogen peroxide to stimulate the development of new capillaries in wound tissue[139]. It is possibly through the production of hydrogen peroxide in the presence of components protecting the cells from oxidative damage that honey is effective in stimulating the rate of healing, and particularly in kick-starting the healing process in wounds that have remained unhealed for a long time.

Another cell growth factor involved in wound healing is the hormone insulin. Wound healing research has shown that intravenous infusion of insulin or applying it to the surface of a wound stimulates the rate of healing[19,89,109]. This is to be expected, as when insulin is present it binds to the insulin receptor protein molecules on the outside of cells and causes them to change conformation, thus triggering a chain of molecular events in the cell that stimulates the uptake of glucose and amino acids, and promotes anabolic metabolism, giving cell growth. The insulin receptor complexes are activated in the same way by low concentrations of hydrogen peroxide[41,72,84], raising the possibility that this is another mechanism by which honey may stimulate wound healing.

Change in the conformation of protein molecules brought about by oxidation by hydrogen peroxide may account for another feature of honey seen when it is used on wounds, that of enzymic debridement of the wound. Although any moist dressing promotes the removal of pus and dead tissue by allowing the action of protein-digesting enzymes in the wound tissues, this debriding action by honey is remarkable. There are two types of protein-digesting enzyme involved in wound tissues: the matrix metalloproteases of the connective tissue[99], and the serine proteases produced by the neutrophil leucocytes[138]. The serine proteases are normally inactive because of the presence of an inhibitor, but hydrogen peroxide inactivates the inhibitor, so the protease becomes active[106]. The metalloproteases are normally present in an inactive conformation, but hydrogen peroxide changes the conformation of these and makes them active[107,148].

CONCLUSIONS

Although honey has in the past been a standard medicine, most medical practitioners in the present day in developed countries are not aware of that, and consider it to be an 'alternative' or 'complementary' medicine. Although there are some very good indications of its effectiveness in reports published in medical journals, there is evidence from randomized controlled clinical trials only for its use as a dressing for burns. Even where there is evidence of effectiveness there is still a reluctance to use alternative medicines where there is no rational explanation for how they work. Thus, it is unlikely that the further randomized controlled clinical trials necessary to conclusively establish the effectiveness of honey as a medicine, and discover how it compares in performance with modern pharmaceuticals will be carried out. This review of the literature has shown that there are rational explanations for the therapeutic effects of honey. But further research is needed to establish that the possible explanations deduced from other biomedical research findings are in fact what is occurring when honey is used.

In any future research, the large variation in composition of honey needs to be taken into account. There has been a tendency in the past to consider any honey to be representative of all honey, and the consequence of this is seen in the very large differences in findings reported on the sensitivity of bacteria to honey[92,93]. In Part 2 of this review mention was made of the awareness of the ancient physicians, and in present day folk medicine, of particular honeys being the best for particular medical uses, yet no account of this is taken in any of the clinical trials of honey. Considerations in the selection of honey for medical use have been discussed[95], and the point raised that until the importance of the anti-inflammatory and antioxidant components of honey have been established, only the antibacterial activity of honey for use as a medicine can be standardized. In light of the likely importance of all of these components, the need for further research to identify their involvement and their nature is needed, so that honeys can be selected to give the best results when used as a medicine.

REFERENCES

1. ABBAS, T (1997) Royal treat. *Living in the Gulf*; pp 50–51.
2. ABUHARFEIL, N; AL-ORAN, R; ABO-SHEHADA, M (1999) The effect of bee honey on the proliferative activity of human B- and T-lymphocytes and the activity of phagocytes. *Food and Agricultural Immunology* 11: 169–177.
3. AGNER, K (1963) Studies on myeloperoxidase activity. 1. Spectrophotometry of the MPO-H2O2 compound. *Acta Chemica Scandinavica* 17(Suppl. 1): S332–S338.
4. AKHTAR, M S; KHAN, M S (1989) Glycaemic responses to three different honeys given to normal and alloxan-diabetic rabbits. *Journal of the Pakistan Medical Association* 39(4): 107–113.
5. AL SOMAI, N; COLEY, K E; MOLAN, P C; HANCOCK, B M (1994) Susceptibility of *Helicobacter pylori* to the antibacterial activity of manuka honey. *Journal of the Royal Society of Medicine* 87(1): 9–12.
6. AL-SWAYEH, O A; ALI, A T M (1998) Effect of ablation of capsaicin-sensitive neurons on gastric protection by honey and sucralfate. *Hepato-Gastroenterology* 45(19): 297–302.
7. ALI, A T M (1995) Natural honey accelerates healing of indomethacin-induced antral ulcers in rats. *Saudi Medical Journal* 16(2): 161–166.
8. ALI, A T M M (1991) Prevention of ethanol-induced gastric lesions in rats by natural honey, and its possible mechanism of action. *Scandinavian Journal of Gastroenterology* 26: 281–288.
9. ALI, A T M M (1995) Natural honey exerts its protective effects against ethanol-induced gastric lesions in rats by preventing depletion of glandular nonprotein sulfhydryls. *Tropical Gastroenterology* 16(1): 18–26.
10. ALI, A T M M; AL-HUMAYYD, M S; MADAN, B R (1990) Natural honey prevents indomethacin- and ethanol-induced gastric lesions in rats. *Saudi Medical Journal* 11(4): 275–279.
11. ALI, A T M M; AL-SWAYEH, O A (1996) The role of nitric oxide in gastric protection by honey. *Saudi Medical Journal* 17: 301–306.
12. ALI, A T M M; AL-SWAYEH, O A (1997) Natural honey prevents ethanol-induced increased vascular permeability changes in the rat stomach. *Journal of Ethnopharmacology* 55(3): 231–238.
13. ALI, A T M M; AL-SWAYEH, O A; AL-HUMAYYD, M S; MUSTAFA, A A; AL-RASHED, R S; AL-TUWAIJIRI, A S (1997) Natural honey prevents ischaemia-reprfusion-induced gastric mucosal lesions and increased vascular permeability in rats. *European Journal of Gastroenterology and Hepatology* 9(11): 1101–1107.
14. ALI, A T M M; CHOWDHURY, M N H; AL HUMAYYD, M S (1991) Inhibitory effect of natural honey on *Helicobacter pylori*. *Tropical Gastroenterology* 12(3): 139–143.
15. ALLEN, K L; MOLAN, P C (1997) The sensitivity of mastitis-causing bacteria to the antibacterial activity of honey. *New Zealand Journal of Agricultural Research* 40: 537–540.
16. ARISTOTLE ((350 BC) 1910) *Historia Animalium*. Oxford University; Oxford, UK.

17. ARMON, P J (1980) The use of honey in the treatment of infected wounds. *Tropical Doctor* 10: 91.
18. BAUER, L; KOHLICH, A; HIRSCHWEHR, R; SIEMANN, U; EBNER, H; SCHEINER, O; KRAFT, D; EBNER, C (1996) Food allergy to honey: pollen or bee products? Characterisation of allergenic proteins in honey by means of immunoblotting. *Journal of Allergy and Clinical Immunology* 97(1): 65–73.
19. BELFIELD, W O; GOLINSKY, S; COMPTON, M D (1970) The use of insulin in open wound healing. *Veterinary Medicine: Small Animal Clinician* 65(5): 455–460.
20. BERGMAN, A; YANAI, J; WEISS, J; BELL, D; DAVID, M P (1983) Acceleration of wound healing by topical application of honey. An animal model. *American Journal of Surgery* 145: 374–376.
21. BLOMFIELD, R (1973) Honey for decubitus ulcers. *Journal of the American Medical Association* 224(6): 905.
22. BLOOMFIELD, E (1976) Old remedies. *Journal of the Royal College of General Practitioners* 26: 576.
23. BOSE, B (1982) Honey or sugar in treatment of infected wounds? *Lancet* i(April 24): 963.
24. BRADY, N F; MOLAN, P C; HARFOOT, C G (1997) The sensitivity of dermatophytes to the antimicrobial activity of manuka honey and other honey. *Pharmaceutical Sciences* 2: 1–3.
25. BRANIKI, F J (1981) Surgery in Western Kenya. *Annals of the Royal College of Surgeons of England* 63: 348–352.
26. BROOKS, F P (1985) The pathophysiology of peptic ulcer disease. *Digestive Diseases and Sciences* 30(11): 15S–29S.
27. BUCKNALL, T E (1984) Factors affecting healing. In T E Bucknall; H Ellis (eds) *Wound healing for surgeon*. Baillière Tindall; London, UK; pp 42–74.
28. BULMAN, M W (1955) Honey as a surgical dressing. *Middlesex Hospital Journal* 55: 188–189.
29. BURDON, R H (1995) Superoxide and hydrogen peroxide in relation to mammalian cell proliferation. *Free Radical Biology and Medicine* 18(4): 775–794.
30. BURLANDO, F (1978) Sull'azione terapeutica del miele nelle ustioni. *Minerva Dermatologica* 113: 699–706.
31. CAVANAGH, D; BEAZLEY, J; OSTAPOWICZ, F (1970) Radical operation for carcinoma of the vulva. A new approach to wound healing. *Journal of Obstetrics and Gynaecology of the British Commonwealth* 77(11): 1037–1040.
32. CHANT, A (1999) The biomechanics of leg ulceration. *Annals of the Royal College of Surgeons of England* 81: 80–85.
33. CHIRIFE, J; HERSZAGE, L; JOSEPH, A; KOHN, E S (1983) *In vitro* study of bacterial growth inhibition in concentrated sugar solutions: microbiological basis for the use of sugar in treating infected wounds. *Antimicrobial Agents and Chemotherapy* 23(5): 766–773.
34. CHUNG, L Y; SCHMIDT, R J; ANDREWS, A M; TURNER, T D (1993) A study of hydrogen peroxide generation by, and antioxidant activity of, Granuflex(tm) (DuoDERM(tm)) Hydrocolloid Granules and some other hydrogel/hydrocolloid wound management materials. *British Journal of Dermatology* 129(2): 145–53.
35. CHURCH, J (1954) Honey as a source of the anti-stiffness factor. *Federation Proceedings of the American Physiology Society* 13(1): 26.
36. COCHRANE, C G (1991) Cellular injury by oxidants. *American Journal of Medicine* 91(Suppl. 3c): 23S–30S.
37. COOPER, R A; MOLAN, P C (1999) The use of honey as an antiseptic in managing Pseudomonas infection. *Journal of Wound Care* 8(4): 161–164.
38. COOPER, R A; MOLAN, P C; HARDING, K G (1999) Antibacterial activity of honey against strains of *Staphylococcus aureus* from infected wounds. *Journal of the Royal Society of Medicine* 92: 283–285.
39. CROSS, C E; HALLIWELL, B; BORISH, E T; PRYOR, W A; AMES, B N; SAUL, R L; MCCORD, J M; HARMAN, D (1987) Oxygen radicals and human disease. *Annals of Internal Medicine* 107: 526–545.
40. CURDA, L; PLOCKOV·, M (1995) Impedance measurement of growth of lactic acid bacteria in dairy cultures with honey addition. *International Dairy Journal* 5: 727–733.
41. CZECH, M P; LAWRENCE JR, J C; LYNN, W S (1974) Evidence for the involvement of sulphydryl oxidation in the regulation of fat cell hexose transport by insulin. *Proceedings of the National Academy of Sciences of the United States of America* 71(10): 4173–4177.
42. DAILEY, L A; IMMING, P (1999) 12-Lipoxygenase: classification, possible therapeutic benefits from inhibition, and inhibitors. *Current Medical Chemistry* 6(5): 389–398.
43. DAVIS, C; ARNOLD, K (1974) Role of meningococal endotoxin in meningococcal purpura. *Journal of Experimental Medicine* 140: 159–171.
44. DEFORGE, L E; FANTONE, J C; KENNEY, J S; REMICK, D G (1992) Oxygen radical scavengers selectively inhibit interleukin 8 production in human whole blood. *Journal of Clinical Investigation* 90: 2123–2129.
45. DOOLEY, C P; COHEN, H (1989) The clinical significance of *Campylobacter pylori*. *Annals of Internal Medicine* 108: 70–79.
46. DUMRONGLERT, E (1983) A follow-up study of chronic wound healing dressing with pure natural honey. *Journal of the National Research Council of Thailand* 15(2): 39–66.
47. DUNFORD, C; COOPER, R A; MOLAN, P C (2000) Using honey as a dressing for infected skin lesions. *Nursing Times* 96(NTPLUS 14): 7–9.
48. DUNFORD, C; COOPER, R A; WHITE, R J; MOLAN, P C (2000) The use of honey in wound management. *Nursing Standard* 15(11): 63–68.
49. EFEM, S E E (1988) Clinical observations on the wound healing properties of honey. *British Journal of Surgery* 75: 679–681.
50. EFEM, S E E (1993) Recent advances in the management of Fournier's gangrene: preliminary observations. *Surgery* 113(2): 200–204.
51. EFEM, S E E; Udoh, K T; Iwara, C I (1992) The antimicrobial spectrum of honey and its clinical significance. *Infection* 20(4): 227–229.
52. EL-BANBY, M; KANDIL, A; ABOU-SEHLY, G; EL-SHERIF, M E; ABDEL-WAHED, K. Healing effect of floral honey and honey from sugar-fed bees on surgical wounds (animal model). In IBRA (eds) *4th International Conference on Apiculture in Tropical Climates, 1989, Cairo*. International Bee Research Association; Cardiff, UK.
53. EL-SUKHON, S N; ABU-HARFEIL, N; SALLAL, A K (1994) Effect of honey on bacterial growth and spore germination. *Journal of Food Protection* 57(10): 918–920.
54. EMARAH, M H (1982) A clinical study of the topical use of bee honey in the treatment of some occular diseases. *Bulletin of Islamic Medicine* 2(5): 422–425.

55. FAROUK, A; HASSAN, T; KASHIF, H; KHALID, S A; MUTAWALI, I; WADI, M (1988) Studies on Sudanese bee honey: laboratory and clinical evaluation. *International Journal of Crude Drug Research* 26(3): 161–168.

56. FLOHÉ, L; BECKMANN, R; GIERTZ, H; LOSCHEN, G (1985) Oxygen-centred free radicals as mediators of inflammation. *In* H Sies (ed) *Oxidative Stress.* Academic Press; London, UK; pp 403–435.

57. FLORIS, I; PROTA, R (1989) Sul miele amaro di Sardegna. *Apicoltore Moderno* 80(2): 55–67.

58. FORDTRAN, J S (1975) Stimulation of active and passive sodium absorption by sugars in the human jejunum. *Journal of Clinical Investigation* 55: 728–737.

59. FOTIDAR, M R; FOTIDAR, S N (1945) 'Lotus' honey. *Indian Bee Journal* 7: 102.

60. FRANKEL, S; ROBINSON, G E; BERENBAUM, M R (1998) Antioxidant capacity and correlated characteristics of 14 unifloral honeys. *Journal of Apicultural Research* 37(1): 27–31.

61. GRIMBLE, G F (1994) Nutritional antioxidants and the modulation of inflammation: theory and practice. *New Horizons* 2(2): 175–185.

62. GUNTHER, R T (1934 (Reprinted 1959)) *The Greek herbal of Dioscorides.* Hafner; New York; 701 pp.

63. GUPTA, S K; SINGH, H; VARSHNEY, A C; PRAKASH, P (1992) Therapeutic efficacy of honey in infected wounds in buffaloes. *Indian Journal of Animal Sciences* 62(6): 521–523.

64. HAFFEJEE, I E; MOOSA, A (1985) Honey in the treatment of infantile gastroenteritis. *British Medical Journal* 290: 1866–1867.

65. HALLIWELL, B; CROSS, C E (1994) Oxygen-derived species: Their relation to human disease and environmental stress. *Environmental Health Perspectives* 102 Suppl 10: 5–12.

66. HARRIS, S (1994) Honey for the treatment of superficial wounds: a case report and review. *Primary Intention* 2(4): 18–23.

67. HASPOLAT, K; BÜYÜKBAS, S; «ENGEL, H (1990) Balin in vitro antibakteriyel ve antifungal etkisi. *Turk Hijiyen ve Deneysel Biyoloji Dergisisi* 47(2): 211–216.

68. HAURY, B; RODEHEAVER, G; VENSKO, J; EDGERTON, M T; EDLICH, R F (1978) Debridement: an essential component of traumatic wound care. *American Journal of Surgery* 135: 238–242.

69. HAYDAK, M H (1955) The nutritional value of honey. *American Bee Journal* 95: 185–191.

70. HEJASE, M J; E., S J; BIHRLE, R; COOGAN, C L (1996) Genital Fournier's gangrene: experience with 38 patients. *Urology* 47(5): 734–739.

71. HELBLING, A; PETER, C; BERCHTOLD, E; BOGDANOV, S; MÜLLER, U (1992) Allergy to honey: relation to pollen and honey bee allergy. *Allergy* 47(1): 41–49.

72. HELM, B A; GUNN, J M (1986) The effect of insulinomimetic agents on protein degradation in H35 hepatoma cells. *Molecular and Cellular Biochemistry* 71(2): 159–166.

73. HUNT, T K; TWOMEY, P; ZEDERFELDT, B; DUNPHY, J E (1967) Respiratory gas tensions and pH in healing wounds. *American Journal of Surgery* 114: 302–307.

74. HUTTON, D J (1966) Treatment of pressure sores. *Nursing Times* 62(46): 1533–1534.

75. HYSLOP, P A; HINSHAW, D B; SCRAUFSTATTER, I U; COCHRANE, C G; KUNZ, S; VOSBECK, K (1995) Hydrogen peroxide as a potent bacteriostatic antibiotic: implications for host defense. *Free Radical Biology and Medicine* 19(1): 31–7.

76. JONES, K P; BLAIR, S; TONKS, A; PRICE, A; COOPER, R (2000) Honey and the stimulation of inflammatory cytokine release from a monocytic cell line. *First World Wound Healing Congress;* Melbourne, Australia.

77. KANDIL, A; EL-BANBY, M; ABDEL-WAHED, K; ABOU-SEHLY, G; EZZAT, N (1987) Healing effect of true floral and false nonfloral honey on medical wounds. *Journal of Drug Research (Cairo)* 17(1–2): 71–75.

78. KATSILAMBROS, N I; PHILIPPIDES, P; TOULIATOU, A; GEORGAKOPOULOS, K; KOFOTZOULI, L; FRANGAKI, D; SISKOUDIS, P; MARANGOS, M; SFIKAKIS, P (1988) Metabolic effects of honey (alone or combined with other foods) in Type II diabetics. *Acta Diabetologica Latina* 25: 197–203.

79. KAUFMAN, T; EICHENLAUB, E H; ANGEL, M F; LEVIN, M; FUTRELL, J W (1985) Topical acidification promotes healing of experimental deep partial thickness skin burns: a randomised double-blind preliminary study. *Burns* 12: 84–90.

80. KAUFMAN, T; LEVIN, M; HURWITZ, D J (1984) The effect of topical hyperalimentation on wound healing rate and granulation tissue formation of experimental deep second degree burns in guinea-pigs. *Burns* 10(4): 252–256.

81. KEAST-BUTLER, J (1980) Honey for necrotic malignant breast ulcers. *Lancet* ii(October 11): 809.

82. KIISTALA, R; HANNUKSELA, M; MÄKINEN-KILJUNEN, S; NIINIMÄKI, A; HAAHTELA, T (1995) Honey allergy is rare in patients sensitive to pollens. *Allergy* 50: 844–847.

83. KLEBANOFF, S J (1980) Myeloperoxidase-mediated cytotoxic systems. *In* A J Sbarra; R R Strauss (eds) *The reticuloendothelial system. A comprehensive treatise. Volume 2. Biochemistry and Metabolism.* Plenum Press; New York; pp 270–308.

84. KOSHIO, O; AKANUMA, Y; KASUGA, M (1988) Hydrogen peroxide stimulates tyrosine phosphorylation of the insulin recepter and its tyrosine kinase activity in intact cells. *Biochemical Journal* 250: 95–101.

85. KUMAR, A; SHARMA, V K; SINGH, H P; PRAKASH, P; SINGH, S P (1993) Efficacy of some indigenous drugs in tissue repair in buffaloes. *Indian Veterinary Journal* 70(1): 42–44.

86. LEVEEN, H H; FALK, G; BOREK, B; DIAZ, C; LYNFIELD, Y; WYNKOOP, B J; MABUNDA, G A; RUBRICUS, J L; CHRISTOUDIAS, G C (1973) Chemical acidification of wounds. An adjuvant to healing and the unfavourable action of alkalinity and ammonia. *Annals of Surgery* 178(6): 745–753.

87. LINEAWEAVER, W; MCMORRIS, S; SOUCY, D; HOWARD, R (1985) Cellular and bacterial toxicities of topical antimicrobials. *Plastic and Reconstructive Surgery* 75(3): 394–396.

88. LINNETT, P, (1996) Honey for equine diarrhoea. *Control and Therapy:* 906.

89. LOPEZ, J E; MENA, B (1968) Local insulin for diabetic gangrene. *Lancet* i: 1199.

90. MCGOVERN, D P B; ABBAS, S Z; VIVIAN, G; DALTON, H R (1999) Manuka honey against *Helicobacter pylori. Journal of the Royal Society of Medicine* 92: 439.

91. MCINERNEY, R J F (1990) Honey – a remedy rediscovered. *Journal of the Royal Society of Medicine* 83: 127.

92. MOLAN, P C (1992) The antibacterial activity of honey. 1. The nature of the antibacterial activity. *Bee World* 73(1): 5–28.

93. MOLAN, P C (1992) The antibacterial activity of honey. 2. Variation in the potency of the antibacterial activity. *Bee World* 73(2): 59–76.
94. MOLAN, P C (1998) A brief review of honey as a clinical dressing. *Primary Intention* 6(4): 148–158.
95. MOLAN, P C (1999) Selection of honey for use as a wound dressing. *Primary Intention* (in press).
96. MOLAN, P C (1999) Why honey is effective as a medicine. 1. Its use in modern medicine. *Bee World* 80(2): 80–92.
97. MOLAN, P C; Allen, K L (1996) The effect of gamma-irradiation on the antibacterial activity of honey. *Journal of Pharmacy and Pharmacology* 48: 1206–1209.
98. MOSSEL, D A A (1980) Honey for necrotic breast ulcers. *Lancet* ii(November 15): 1091.
99. MURPHY, G; REYNOLDS, J J; BRETZ, U; BAGGIOLINI, M (1982) Partial purification of collagenase and gelatinase from human polymorphonuclear leukocytes. *Biochemical Journal* 203: 209–221.
100. MURRELL, G A C; FRANCIS, M J O; BROMLEY, L (1990) Modulation of fibroblast proliferation by oxygen free radicals. *Biochemical Journal* 265: 659–665.
101. NDAYISABA, G; BAZIRA, L; HABONIMANA, E; MUTEGANYA, D (1993) Clinical and bacteriological results in wounds treated with honey. *Journal of Orthopaedic Surgery* 7(2): 202–204.
102. NIINIKOSKI, J; KIVISAARI, J; VILJANTO, J (1977) Local hyperalimentation of experimental granulation tissue. *Acta Chiropida Scandinavica* 143: 201–206.
103. NYCHAS, G J; DILLON, V M; BOARD, R G (1988) Glucose, the key substrate in the microbiological changes in meat and certain meat products. *Biotechnology and Applied Biochemistry* 10: 203–231.
104. OBI, C L; UGOJI, E O; EDUN, S A; LAWAL, S F; ANYIWO, C E (1994) The antibacterial effect of honey on diarrhoea causing bacterial agents isolated in Lagos, Nigeria. *African Journal of Medical Sciences* 23: 257–260.
105. ORYAN, A; ZAKER, S R (1998) Effects of topical application of honey on cutaneous wound healing in rabbits. *Journal of Veterinary Medicine, Series A* 45(3): 181–188.
106. OSSANNA, P J; TEST, S T; MATHESON, N R; REGIANI, S; WEISS, S J (1986) Oxidative regulation of neutrophil elastase-alpha-1-proteinase inhibitor interactions. *Journal of Clinical Investigation* 77: 1939–1951.
107. PEPPIN, G J; WEISS, S J (1986) Activation of the endogenous metalloproteinase, gelatinase, by triggered human neutrophils. *Proceedings of the National Academy of Sciences of the United States of America* 83: 4322–4326.
108. PHUAPRADIT, W; SAROPALA, N (1992) Topical application of honey in treatment of abdominal wound disruption. *Australian and New Zealand Journal of Obstetrics and Gynaecology* 32(4): 381–384.
109. PIERRE, E J; BARROW, R E; HAWKINS, H K; NGUYEN, T T; SAKURAI, Y; DESAI, M; WOLFE, R R; HERNDON, D N (1998) Effects of insulin on wound healing. *Journal of Trauma, Injury, Infection and Critical Care* 44(2): 342–345.
110. POSTMES, T; BOGAARD, A E VAN DEN; HAZEN, M (1993) Honey for wounds, ulcers, and skin graft preservation. *Lancet* 341(8847): 756–757.
111. POSTMES, T; BOGAARD, A E VAN DEN; HAZEN, M (1995) The sterilization of honey with cobalt 60 gamma radiation: a study of honey spiked with *Clostridium botulinum* and *Bacillus subtilis*. *Experentia (Basel)* 51: 986–989.
112. POSTMES, T; VANDEPUTTE, J (1999) Recombinant growth factors or honey? *Burns* 25(7): 676–678.
113. POSTMES, T J; BOSCH, M M C; DUTRIEUX, R; BAARE, J VAN; HOEKSTRA, M J (1997) Speeding up the healing of burns with honey. An experimental study with histological assessment of wound biopsies. *In* A Mizrahi; Y Lensky (eds) *Bee products: properties, applications and apitherapy*. Plenum Press; New York; pp 27–37.
114. PRUITT, K M; REITER, B (1985) Biochemistry of peroxidase system: antimicrobial effects. *In* K M Pruitt; J O Tenovuo (eds) *The lactoperoxidase system: chemistry and biological significance*. Marcel Dekker; New York; pp 144–178.
115. ROOS, D (1991) The respiratory burst of phagocytic leucocytes. *Drug Investigation* 3(suppl. 2): 48–53.
116. ROTH, L A; KWAN, S; SPORNS, P (1986) Use of a disc-assay system to detect oxytetracycline residues in honey. *Journal of Food Protection* 49(6): 436–441.
117. RYAN, G B; MAJNO, G (1977) *Inflammation*. Upjohn; Kalamazoo, Michigan, USA; 80 pp.
118. SAÏSSY, J M; GUIGNARD, B; PATS, B; GUIAVARCH, M; ROUVIER, B (1995) Pulmonary edema after hydrogen peroxide irrigation of a war wound. *Intensive Care Medicine* 21(3): 287–288.
119. SALAHUDEEN, A K; CLARK, E C; NATH, K A (1991) Hydrogen peroxide-induced renal injury. A protective role for pyruvate *in vitro* and *in vivo*. *Journal of Clinical Investigation* 88(6): 1886–1893.
120. SAMANTA, A; BURDEN, A C; JONES, G R (1985) Plasma glucose responses to glucose, sucrose, and honey in patients with diabetes mellitus: an analysis of glycaemic and peak incremental indices. *Diabetic Medicine* 2(5): 371–373.
121. SCHRECK, R; RIEBER, P; BAEUERLE, P A (1991) Reactive oxygen intermediates as apparently widely used messengers in the activation of the NF-kB transcription factor and HIV-1. *EMBO Journal* 10(8): 2247–2258.
122. SHEIKH, D; SHAMS-UZ-ZAMAN; NAQVI, S B; SHEIKH, M R; ALI, G (1995) Studies on the antimicrobial activity of honey. *Pakistan Journal of Pharmaceutical Sciences* 8(1): 51–62.
123. SILVER, I A (1980) The physiology of wound healing. *In* T K Hunt (ed) *Wound healing and wound infection: theory and surgical practice*. Appleton-Century-Crofts; New York; pp 11–28.
124. SILVETTI, A N (1981) An effective method of treating long-enduring wounds and ulcers by topical applications of solutions of nutrients. *Journal of Dermatolology, Surgery and Oncology* 7(6): 501–508.
125. SIMON, R H; SCOGGIN, C H; PATTERSON, D (1981) Hydrogen peroxide causes the fatal injury to human fibroblasts exposed to oxygen radicals. *Journal of Biological Chemistry* 256(14): 7181–7186.
126. SINCLAIR, R D; RYAN, T J (1994) Proteolytic enzymes in wound healing: the role of enzymatic debridement. *Australasian Journal of Dermatology* 35: 35–41.
127. SOMERFIELD, S D (1991) Honey and healing. *Journal of the Royal Society of Medicine* 84(3): 179.
128. SUBRAHMANYAM, M (1991) Topical application of honey in treatment of burns. *British Journal of Surgery* 78(4): 497–498.
129. SUBRAHMANYAM, M (1993) Honey impregnated gauze versus polyurethane film (OpSite(r)) in the treatment of burns – a prospective randomised study. *British Journal of Plastic Surgery* 46(4): 322–323.
130. SUBRAHMANYAM, M (1994) Honey-impregnated gauze versus amniotic membrane in the treatment of burns. *Burns* 20(4): 331–333.

131. SUBRAHMANYAM, M (1996) Honey dressing versus boiled potato peel in the treatment of burns: a prospective randomized study. *Burns* 22(6): 491–493.

132. SUBRAHMANYAM, M (1998) A prospective randomised clinical and histological study of superficial burn wound healing with honey and silver sulfadiazine. *Burns* 24(2): 157–161.

133. SUGUNA, L; CHANDRAKASAN, G; RAMAMOORTHY, U; THOMAS JOSEPH, K (1993) Influence of honey on biochemical and biophysical parameters of wounds in rats. *Journal of Clinical Biochemistry and Nutrition* 14: 91–99.

134. SUGUNA, L; CHANDRAKASAN, G; THOMAS JOSEPH, K (1992) Influence of honey on collagen metabolism during wound healing in rats. *Journal of Clinical Biochemistry and Nutrition* 13: 7–12.

135. SWAIM, S F (1980) *Surgery of traumatized skin: management and reconstruction in the dog and cat.* W B Saunders Co.; Philadelphia, USA; 120–122 pp.

136. TANAKA, H; HANUMADASS, M; MATSUDA, H; SHIMAZAKI, S; WALTER, R J; MATSUDA, T (1995) Hemodynamic effects of delayed initiation of antioxidant therapy (beginning two hours after burn) in extensive third-degree burns. *Journal of Burn Care and Rehabilitation* 16(6): 610–615.

137. TATNALL, F M; LEIGH, I M; GIBSON, J R (1991) Assay of antiseptic agents in cell culture: conditions affecting cytotoxicity. *Journal of Hospital Infection* 17(4): 287–296.

138. TONNESEN, M G; WORTHEN, G S; JOHNSTON, R B JR. (1988) Neutrophil emigration, activation and tissue damage. In R A F Clark; P M Henson (eds) *The molecular and cellular biology of wound repair.* Plenum Press; New York, London; pp 149–183.

139. TUR, E; BOLTON, L; CONSTANTINE, B E (1995) Topical hydrogen peroxide treatment of ischemic ulcers in the guinea pig: Blood recruitment in multiple skin sites. *Journal of the American Academy of Dermatology* 33(2 Pt 1): 217–221.

140. TURNER, F J (1983) *Hydrogen peroxide and other oxidant disinfectants.* Lea & Febiger; Philadelphia, USA; 240–250 pp.

141. VARDI, A; BARZILAY, Z; LINDER, N; COHEN, H A; PARET, G; BARZILAI, A (1998) Local application of honey for treatment of neonatal postoperative wound infection. *Acta Paediatrica* 87(4): 429–432.

142. VILJANTO, J; RAEKALLIO, J (1976) Local hyperalimentation of open wounds. *British Journal of Surgery* 63: 427–430.

143. WADI, M; AL-AMIN, H; FAROUQ, A; KASHEF, H; KHALED, S A (1987) Sudanese bee honey in the treatment of suppurating wounds. *Arab Medico* 3: 16–18.

144. WAHDAN, H A L (1998) Causes of the antimicrobial activity in honey. *Infection* 36(1): 30–35.

145. WAKHLE, D M; DESAI, D B (1991) Estimation of antibacterial activity of some Indian honeys. *Indian Bee Journal* 53(1–4): 80–90.

146. WEBER, H (1937) Honig zur Behandlung vereiterter Wunden. *Therapie der Gegenwart* 78: 547.

147. WEHEIDA, S M; NAGUBIB, H H; EL-BANNA, H M; MARZOUK, S (1991) Comparing the effects of two dressing techniques on healing of low grade pressure ulcers. *Journal of the Medical Research Institute, Alexandria University* 12(2): 259–278.

148. WEISS, S J; PEPPIN, G; ORTIZ, X; RAGSDALE, C; TEST, S T (1985) Oxidative autoactivation of latent collagenase by human neutrophils. *Science* 227: 747–749.

149. WHITE, J W (1975) Composition of honey. In E Crane (ed) *Honey: a comprehensive survey.* Heinemann; London, UK; pp 157–206.

150. WILLIX, D J; MOLAN, P C; HARFOOT, C J (1992) A comparison of the sensitivity of wound-infecting species of bacteria to the antibacterial activity of manuka honey and other honey. *Journal of Applied Bacteriology* 73: 388–394.

151. WINTER, G D (1962) Formation of the scab and the rate of epithelialization of superficial wounds in the skin of the young domestic pig. *Nature (London)* 193(4812): 293–294.

152. WOOD, B; RADEMAKER, M; MOLAN, P C (1997) Manuka honey, a low cost leg ulcer dressing. *New Zealand Medical Journal* 110: 107.

153. WORLD HEALTH ORGANISATION (1976) *Treatment and prevention of dehydration in diarrhoeal diseases.* WHO; 31 pp.

154. YANG, K L (1944) The use of honey in the treatment of chilblains, non-specific ulcers, and small wounds. *Chinese Medical Journal* 62: 55–60.

155. ZAIß (1934) Der Honig in äußerlicher Anwendung. *Münchener Medizinische Wochenschrift* (49): 1891–1893.

PETER MOLAN

Honey Research Unit, Department of Biological Sciences, University of Waikato, Hamilton, New Zealand

How does honey heal wounds?

ROSE COOPER

INTRODUCTION

Mankind has always needed wound remedies. In ancient civilisations the benefits of local animal, plant and mineral resources in concoctions applied to wounds must have been learnt by trial and error, and accumulated wisdom disseminated by word of mouth. Vestiges of that knowledge are still utilized in folk medicine. Documented evidence that honey was used in wound remedies dates from approximately 2500 BC[1], and can be intermittently traced to conventional medical practice until the middle of the twentieth century. Modern wound management was revolutionized by the advent of antibiotics during the 1950s, and later by the development of sophisticated, innovative dressing materials designed to maintain a moist healing environment. In conventional medicine these improvements, coupled with a transition to evidence-based clinical practice lead to the discontinuation of many empirical therapies. Honey lost favour because the evidence supporting its efficacy in wound treatment was largely anecdotal. Even though many modern physicians remain sceptical, claims that honey has important benefits in wound care continue to accumulate[2]. Until the successful elucidation of mechanisms at a cellular and molecular level, and the collection of objective data derived from randomized controlled clinical trials, speculation about the role of honey in wound healing will continue. In the meantime, reviewing the normal healing process and the reasons why wounds fail to heal, might provide an insight into the ways in which honey might influence the healing process.

NORMAL WOUND HEALING

Wounds result from many different deliberate and unintentional actions. All wounds are unique, varying in size, shape, position and cause, but all wounds involve the death of epithelial cells, loss of blood, tissue damage, and the disruption of physical barriers that normally prevent infection. Healing restores tissue integrity following injury and, fortunately, many wounds proceed to heal without difficulty. The normal healing process involves a complex sequence of events whose control mechanisms are not yet fully elucidated. A sequence of three overlapping phases can be identified: inflammation, cell proliferation and tissue remodelling[3]. Because wounding breaches the first line of defence, a rapid reaction is initiated as part of the normal survival response. Damage to blood vessels allows the release of blood immediately after wounding, and allows platelets to adhere to endothelial basement membrane as well as strands of elastin and collagen that are embedded in connective tissue. Platelet adhesion leads to the formation of platelet aggregates that cause the release of stored proteins, which activate a complex sequence of protein reactions. These in turn result in the formation of a fragile matrix of loose protein fibres known as a fibrin clot. Blood cells become trapped within this mesh forming a sticky plug that prevents further bleeding. It also helps to loosely hold together the severed ends of blood vessels and to minimize acquisition of contamination from external sources.

The duration of the inflammatory phase is variable, but usually lasts for 3 days, and can be sub-divided into early and late stages. The formation of a blood clot within the wounded area helps to re-establish homeostasis. Cellular and tissue damage initiates a complex local response where soluble chemical signals that are released, regulate the movement of cells into the injured site, and their activity on arrival. Acute inflammation is characterized by the dilation of blood vessels with increased permeability allowing the movement of fluid and cells into the injured site, causing swelling and increased pain. Initially neutrophils together with relatively low numbers of monocytes are attracted. Neutrophil infiltration facilitates the removal of damaged cells and contaminating microorganisms by phagocytosis. Later, numbers of monocytes exceed neutrophils, and fibroblasts are recruited. Cells invading into the provisional matrix provided by the fibrin clot are stimulated to divide. Within the wound tissue monocytes differentiate into macrophages and gradually become activated to synthesize a cocktail of growth factors and cytokines that controls the later stages of the healing process[3,4]. Macrophages continue to remove micro-organisms, tissue debris and exhausted neutrophils by phagocytosis. Fibroblasts are stimulated to synthesize components of the extracellular matrix (such as collagen, fibronectin and proteoglycans).

Approximately 12 hours after wounding, epidermal cells are stimulated to divide. Initially these cells move over one another towards the incisional wound space, but once migrating cells make contact with one another, migration ceases and continued cell division leads to thickening of the epidermal cell layer.

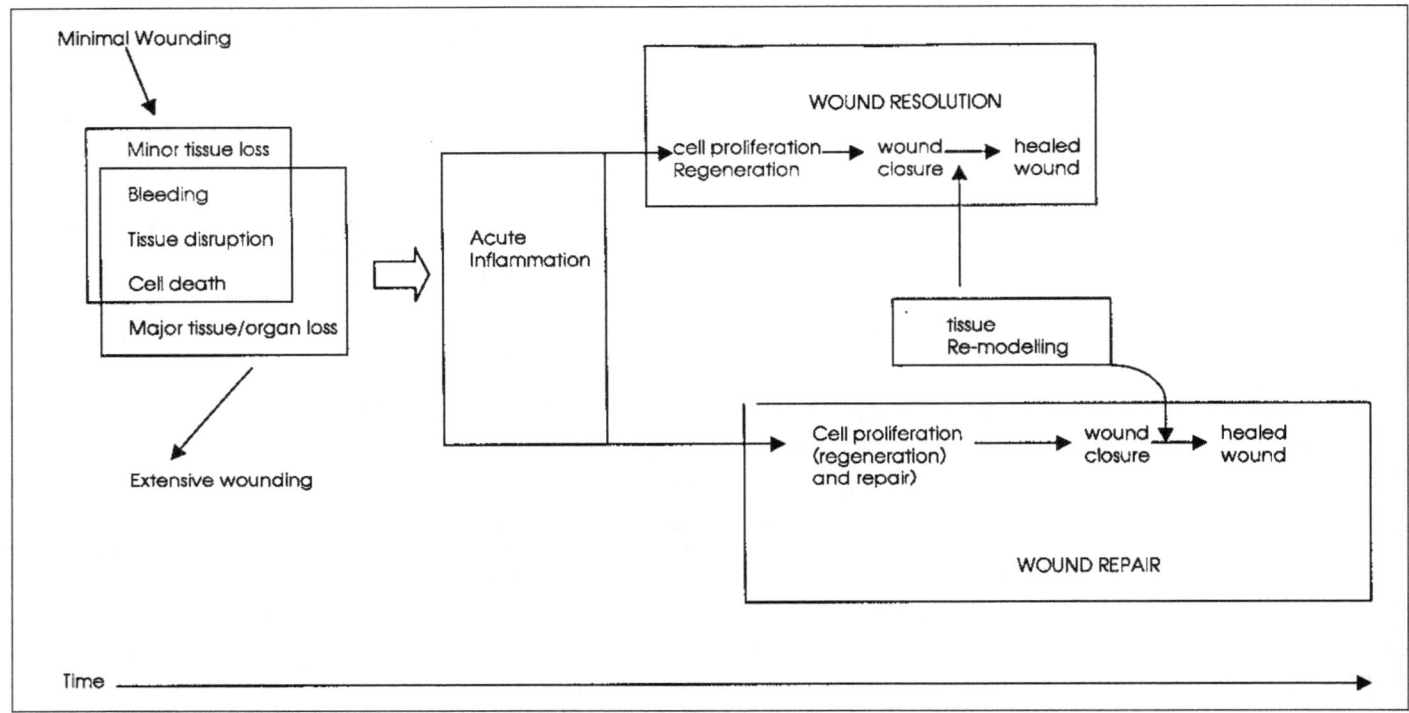

Normal wound healing.

Towards the close of the inflammatory phase, angiogenesis (the formation of new capillaries) is initiated; buds extend from existing capillaries and elongate to form new capillaries. As the inflammatory phase continues, the fibrin clot becomes progressively replaced by neutrophils, macrophages, fibroblasts, newly synthesized extracellular material and capillaries, whilst being solubilized by a proteolytic enzyme. The resultant tissue is known as granulation tissue, and marks the transition to the proliferative phase.

During the proliferative phase, continued division of activated fibroblasts and collagen deposition contributes to wound repair. Transformation of fibroblasts to myofibroblasts allows continued synthesis of extracellular matrix components, followed by wound contraction. Continued development of capillaries within granulation tissue is essential for effective fibroblast function, but once the cavity of a wound has been restored and re-epithelialization is complete the maturation stage commences. Late in the proliferative stage leukocytes are attracted to the site of a wound, and the inflammatory infiltrate is replaced, swelling diminishes and recent vasculature reduces. The extent of the proliferative phase on average is between 5 and 14 days; it precedes the maturation, phase, which can extend to one year's duration. During maturation tissue remodelling contributes to the re-establishment of normal tensile strength and the modification of scar tissue. Regression of capillaries formed during the inflammatory phase continues and regeneration of dermal structures is completed, where possible.

Events in the wound following acute inflammation are influenced by the extent of the injury, and by the cause of the insult. When damage is minimal cell proliferation usually allows restoration of tissue with normal organization and minimal scarring. Stem cells are essential for the restoration of epidermal and dermal integrity[6]. These multipotent cells are located in hair follicles and have the potential to give rise to all types of cell within the epidermis, sebaceous glands and hair follicles. When extensive loss of tissue has occurred during wounding, loss of stem cells means that res-

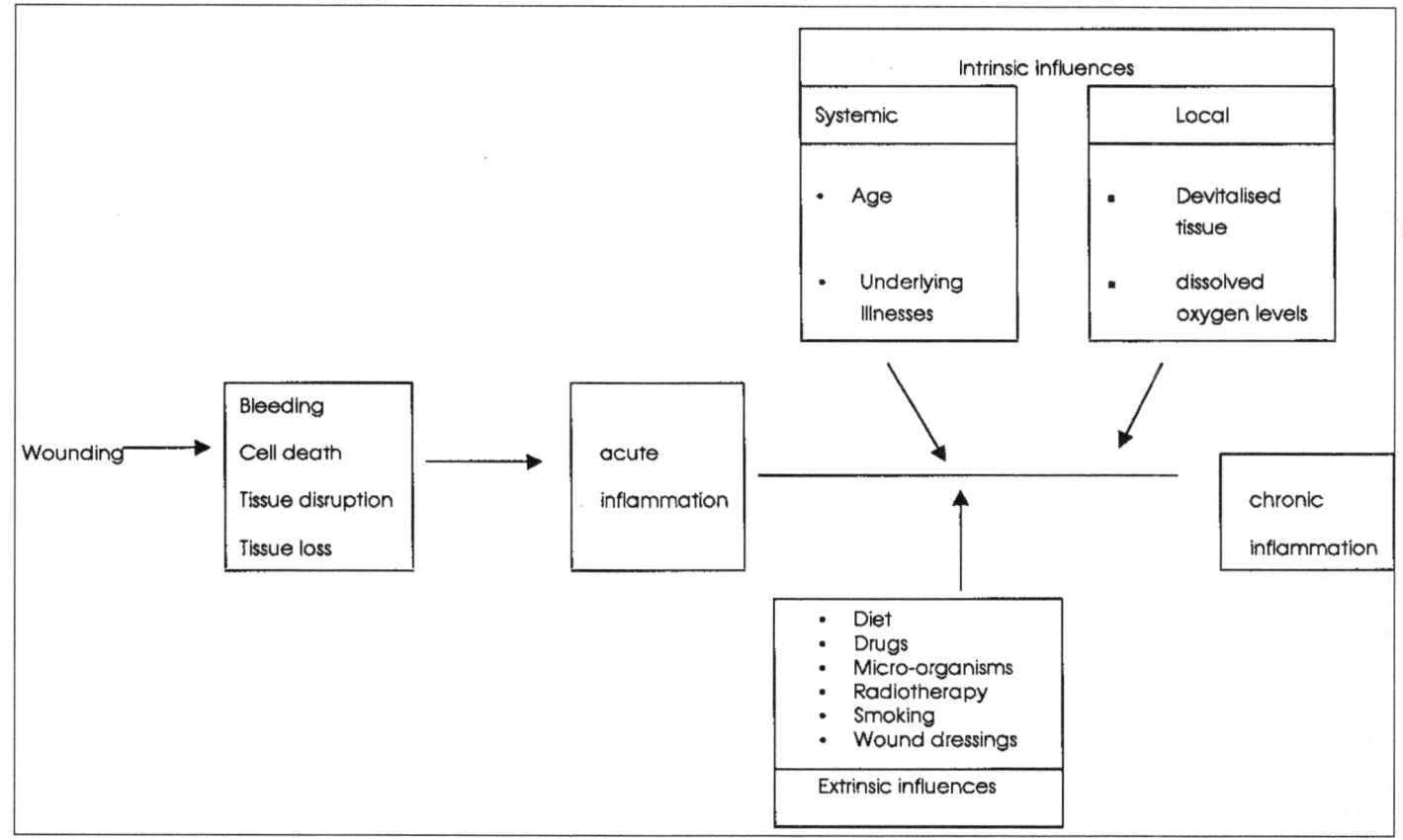

Factors that contribute to delayed healing.

toration of normal tissue organization is not achievable because some cells (e.g. nerve and striated muscle) are unable to divide, and cannot regenerate. These cells are, therefore, not restored during healing. Hence cell proliferation during the proliferative and maturation phases of healing leads to tissue replacement rather than cell restoration (or regeneration). Specialized organization may be lost and wound repair rather than wound resolution results.

Failure to heal

The reasons why wounds fail to heal are complex and diverse. The size, shape, location and cause of a wound allows decisions to be formulated on appropriate wound management strategies, and predictions to be made on the time frames expected to achieve successful healing. Acute wounds are characterized by relatively minor tissue loss and short predicted healing times. If wound margins are entire and closure is possible, rapid healing proceeds by primary intention. Where tissue loss is more extensive and wound margins are widely separated, healing proceeds more slowly by secondary intention. Chronic wounds fail to heal at predicted rates, and instead of a transition from the acute inflammatory phase into the proliferative phase, a transition into chronic inflammation occurs. Normal wound healing is a tightly regulated dynamic process in which the activity of several cell types, the extracellular matrix, soluble growth factors and cytokines is precisely co-ordinated. Many influences, both internal and external, can impinge on this process, altering timing and progression from acute inflammation to proliferation and maturation phases of normal healing.

Intrinsic factors that affect wound healing

Internal influences on the wound healing process can be divided into those that relate to the patient as a whole (systemic) and those that relate to a wound in particular (local). Older patients usually heal more slowly than younger ones, with alterations in the inflammatory response, retarded angiogenesis, reduced collagen synthesis and turnover, and delayed epithelialization[7]. The presence of underlying disease in a patient can compromise wound healing. Impaired renal function affects fluid and electrolyte balance, and blood coagulation pathways. Because ureamia restricts cell growth and division, formation of granulation tissue is reduced, fibroblast activity is depressed and collagen synthesis decreased. Hence the tensile strength of a wound is lowered.

Diabetes mellitus is the disease that probably has the most significant impact on wound healing. Although there is not yet a complete explanation of the pathogenesis of this disease in the impairment of healing, several influences have been identified: peripheral vascular disease, decreased immuno-competency and peripheral neuropathy[8]. Hardening and thickening of blood vessels is often observed in diabetic patients, especially in their limbs. Following injury, local blood supply is necessary for an adequate supply of oxygen, nutrients and inflammatory cells, but, the function of neutrophils that infiltrate the wounds of diabetic patients is impaired with respect to their migratory responses, adherence, cytokine production and bactericidal activity. Furthermore, the lymphocytes that invade at a later stage also demonstrate impaired function and cytokine synthesis. Hence the wounds of diabetic patients have a tendency not only to delayed healing, but also increased prevalence of infection. Such wounds are likely to become chronic wounds. Within the milieu of the wound, dissolved oxygen levels are critical for successful healing: tissues without effective blood supply (ischaemic) fail to heal normally. Yet the role of oxygen in healing is not fully elucidated and there are indications that different levels are required at different stages. Macrophages require low levels of dissolved oxygen (hypoxia) to promote angiogenesis[9], but fibroblasts require oxygen to synthesize collagen[10].

Another intrinsic factor that inhibits wound healing is the presence of necrotic tissue and eschar. Removal of this material is facilitated by leucocytes and macrophages with proteolytic enzymes and phagocytosis. The natural process can be accelerated by applying hydrocolloid dressings that maintain a moist environment; excessive amounts can be removed surgically and application of exogenous proteolytic enzymes also promotes rapid debridement.

TABLE 1. Potential wound pathogens.

Gram positive facultative cocci

β-haemolytic streptococci
  Streptococcus pyogenes
  Streptococcus species (Group G)
  coagulase negative staphylococci
  Staphylococcus epidermidis

enterococci
  Enterococcus faecium
  Enterococcus faecalis

Staphylococci
  Staphylococcus aureus
  Methicillin-resistant *Staphylococcus aureus* (MRSA)

Gram negative aerobic rods

  Pseudomonas aeruginosa

Gram negative facultative rods

  Acinetobacter spp.
  Enterobacter spp.
  Escherichia coli
  Klebsiella spp.
  Proteus spp.
  Serratia marescens

Anaerobes

  Bacteroides spp.
  Clostridium spp.
  Peptostreptococcus spp.
  Prevotella spp.

Fungi

yeasts
  Candida spp.

mycelial fungi
  Aspergillus spp.
  Fusarium spp.

Extrinsic factors that affect wound healing

The importance of diet has often been under-estimated, even though malnutrition has multiple effects on healing by decreasing the inflammatory response, reducing collagen synthesis and decreasing the deposition of extracellular matrix[11]. Essential dietary components required for effective healing include amino acids, vitamins A, C and E, zinc, copper, iron and trace elements.

A number of therapeutic agents that are used for cancer patients, transplant recipients and victims of inflammatory diseases have deleterious effects on wound healing. These drugs function by inhibiting protein synthesis, blocking cell division or dampening the inflammatory responses, and therefore induce multiple adverse effects on healing.

Radiotherapy also has serious consequences on healing, because actively dividing cells are easily killed by radiation and the development of new capillaries is impeded. An irradiated wound may, therefore, become an ischaemic wound. The presence of foreign bodies (such as glass, metal, wood, plastic, soil) always inhibits healing, and removal by debridement is imperative for healing to continue.

The most significant extrinsic factor that impinges on wound healing is the presence of micro-organisms. Although a consensus on the impact of specific micro-organisms on the healing process is not yet agreed, the development of an infection causes serious delays in healing. The skin and mucosa provide physical barriers against infection, but injury destroys the integrity of barriers and allows the ingress of micro-organisms to vulnerable tissues from the environment, surrounding skin or from other body sites. The fate of those intruders depends on the interaction of a multitude of host and microbial factors. Many organisms will be removed by phagocytosis, and some will fail to survive because they are not suitably adapted for the wound environment. Those organisms that persist may either colonize or infect the wound. Many wounds support mixed communities of microbial species, but antimicrobial strategies are only indicated when infection develops or when wounds colonized by destructive bacteria (β-haemolytic streptococci or pseudomonads) require skin grafts. Many species have the potential to cause wound infections (table 1). In addition to delaying healing, infection can lead to pain, swelling, malodours and wound dehiscence. Microbial colonization of wounds has conflicting implications. Some studies have failed to associate specific micro-organisms with delayed healing[13,14] whereas *Pseudomonas* and *Proteus* have been recovered from enlarging and necrotic lesions[15], *Pseudomonas aeruginosa* has been linked to larger wounds[16] and *Staphylococcus aureus* and β-haemolytic streptococci associated with delayed healing[16]. French military surgeons first recognized that even low numbers of β-haemolytic streptococci were a contra-indication to healing by primary intention[17], and plastic surgeons in the 1950s recognized the destructive nature of β-haemolytic streptococci to skin grafts[18]. The significance of β-haemolytic streptococci in causing failure of skin grafts to chronic leg ulcers has recently been

---

TABLE 2 : Curative Properties of honey.

Antibacterial activity
- inhibition of potential wound pathogens
- sanitization of offensive smells

Anti-inflammatory properties
- resolution of oedema
- reduction of pain

Stimulation of rapid healing
- stimulation of phagocytosis and debridement
- stimulation of angiogenesis
- promotion of granulation tissue formation
- cell proliferation
- collagen synthesis
- re-epithelialization

TABLE 3. Minimum Inhibition Concentrations (% v/v) of honey for bacteria isolated from infected wounds[27].

Organism Pasture	Number of strains tested	Artificial honey		Manuka honey
			honey	
Enterococcus faecalis	4	28.6	6.6	8.4
Escherichia coli	4	23.4	4.0	7.8
Klebsiella oxytoca	2	27.8	3.7	7.5
MRSA	3	>30	2.3	2.9
Proteus mirabilis	1	28.6	5.2	6.3
Proteus morganii	3	22.8	3.6	5.1

reinforced and antimicrobial therapy advocated to ensure their removal before grafting[19].

THE CURATIVE PROPERTIES OF HONEY

Honey is claimed to have diverse curative properties in wounds (table 2). The evidence to support these claims has already been comprehensively reviewed[2,20,21,22]. To avoid unnecessary repetition, it is intended here to highlight only recent reports that extend our understanding of the role of honey in promoting wound healing. Antibacterial properties of honey are potentially beneficial to healing by controlling wound infections or by inhibiting deleterious wound colonizations. Anti-inflammatory effects of honey have several possible advantages in healing. High osmolarity favours the outflow of fluid from wound tissue, helping to relieve oedema and pain. Hence movement of fluid from underlying tissues and capillaries in response to this osmotic pull will lead to improvements in microcirculation and increased levels of dissolved oxygen and nutrients. Additional effects on free radical formation and fibroblast activity have been explained[2].

Any improvement in the quality of life for a patient, such as the sanitation of offensive wound smells or the relief of pain, may not directly advance the healing process, but more subtle indirect effects on patients' attitudes cannot be discounted.

Whether honey can ameliorate the intrinsic factors that retard wound healing is questionable. Patients with underlying disease, ischaemic wounds, advanced age or on certain therapeutic regimes are especially disadvantaged. However, improved debridement is often reported when honey is applied to wounds[2]. This reflects activation of macrophages and represents an important intrinsic factor with realistic potential for improvement.

Recent evidence that honey influences wound healing

The evidence that honey affects wound healing is based on observations derived from three sources: *in vitro* studies, animal models and clinical data[2,20,21,22]. Much of that evidence relies on monitoring the effects of honey on wounds in animals, or in patients and does not adequately explain at a molecular level how honey modulates the function of cells, extracellular components and mediating molecules. Antibacterial activity, however, has been extensively investigated *in vitro* and *in vivo*.

Recent evidence of antibacterial properties

In 1992 seventy-seven microbial species were reported to be inhibited by honey[23]. Unfortunately published sensitivities were inconsistent because honeys of unspecified origin and unknown potency were utilized; when honeys of known floral source and specified potency were used, a more meaningful pattern of inhibition emerged. Willix et al.[24] showed that seven wound pathogens were inhibited by a high peroxide pasture honey and a non-peroxide manuka honey (both of median level potency) at concentrations below 11% (v/v). Because the bacteria tested in this study were type cultures rather than clinical isolates, relevance to clinical practice was dubious. Similar honeys were used to test the sensitivity of 20 strains of *Pseudomonas aeruginosa*[25] and 58 strains of *Staphylococcus aureus*[26] isolated from infected wounds. Minimum inhibition concentrations (MIC) of manuka (non-peroxide) and pasture honey (hydrogen peroxide) against *P. aeruginosa* were 6.9% (v/v) and 7.1% (v/v), respectively, and against *S. aureus* were 2.9% (v/v) and 3.8%(v/v), respectively. Using similar methodology[25,26], the sensitivity of a more extensive range of wound pathogens has now been tested (table 3). An artificial honey[27] was included here to determine the extent of bacterial inhibition attributable to sugar content. None of the wound pathogens tested were inhibited by artificial honey incorporated into agar plates at less than 22% (v/v), whereas inhibition was observed with manuka and pasture honey at concentrations below 10% (v/v). Osmolarity alone, therefore, does not explain inhibition of these species. Similar sensitivity of β-haemolytic streptococci and vancomycin resistant enterococci to the same honeys has been observed (unpublished data). Except for anaerobes, most bacteria capable of causing wound infection, or capable of delaying wound healing by colonization, have now been shown to be inhibited by two median potency honeys at concentrations below 10% (v/v) in laboratory tests. Hence honey diluted by a factor of at least 10 is capable of preventing growth of many potential wound pathogens.

When applied to wounds, honey will be diluted by exuded body fluids; whether its inhibitory properties are retained *in vivo* can be gauged from clinical observations. There are many reports that wounds treated with honey become sterile within 7 to 10 days[2,20,21,22], although personal observations have not always confirmed this conclusion (unpublished data). Nevertheless, honey caused the eradication of *Enterococcus* species and *P. aeruginosa* from multiple, infected, non-healing leg lesions caused by meningococcal septicaemia[28], with simultaneous loss of offensive smell and reduction in pain[28]. The most noticeable effect of using honey-impregnated dressings on this patient was the rapid formation of granulation tissue, which marked the transition from chronic inflammation to wound repair, followed by the clearance of infection. Signs of epithelialization were noticed within several days, although enterococci and pseudomonads were eliminated after several weeks, and *S. aureus* persisted throughout the healing process. Hence infection was not exclusively responsible for failure to heal in this patient. Honey was able to stimulate healing as well as clearing infection.

Inhibition of MRSA (methicillin-resistant *S. aureus*) in chronic wounds has recently been reported[29,30]. In one patient[30] healing was compromised by immuno-suppression following liver transplantation, and by hydroxyurea therapy for a myeloproliferative disorder. Conventional therapies had failed to heal this ulcer, yet topical application of manuka honey achieved eradication of MRSA within two weeks, and wound closure was completed one week later. Hydroxyurea is believed to have induced the formation of the ulcer by damaging basal keratinocytes and collagen synthesis; the immuno-suppressant (cyclosporin) compounded the situation by adversely affecting collagen deposition. Colonization by sub-clinical levels of MRSA is unlikely to have precluded healing in this ulcer, and it is remarkable that rapid healing was achieved by manuka honey without cessation of either hydroxyurea or cyclosporin.

CONCLUSION

Honey is considered by some to be a 'worthless but harmless substance'[31], but this is confounded by an impressive array of observations that supports the efficacy of this ancient remedy in modern wound care. Unfortunately, most of these examples were derived from single case studies, small cohort studies or from a small number of comparative clinical trials. At present there is no definitive data that has been derived from double-blind randomized controlled clinical trials. Also, the accumulated evidence mainly relates to observed secondary effects such as the inhibition of wound pathogens, anti-inflammatory activity, stimulation of granulation tissue formation, or rapid cell proliferation and re-epithelialization. Whereas those effects undoubtedly contribute towards progression in the healing process, the mechanisms by which those effects were caused have not been elucidated. Healing is a dynamic process that involves the integrated function of blood components, extracellular matrix and several different cell types. The temporal and spatial organization of each of these contributors is delicately regulated by cellular marker molecules and soluble mediators generated in a coordinated way by cells involved in both the degradative and reparative stages of healing. Soluble molecules (growth factors and cytokines) bind specifically to the surface of their respective target cells and thereby trigger intracellular signals that modulate the growth, division and/or activity of each target cell.

Because cells activated in this way in turn produce molecules that affect other cell types, a complex sequence of events ensues, and perturbations that affect their production have profound effects. Clearly there is a need to investigate processes at a molecular and cellular level, and to be able to demonstrate which components of honey elicit specific cell responses that advance healing. A start on this approach has been made[32]. Until the events of normal wound healing are fully explained, and the control points that limit healing are fully understood, a detailed explanation of the role of honey in promoting healing might remain obscure. In the meantime, there is much research to be undertaken.

REFERENCES

1. JONES, H R (2001) Honey and healing through the ages. *In* Munn, P A (ed) *Honey and healing.* IBRA; Cardiff, UK; pp 1–4.
2. MOLAN, P C (2001) Why honey is effective as a medicine. *In* Munn, P A (ed) *Honey and healing.* IBRA; Cardiff, UK; pp 5–13, 14–26.
3. CLARKE, R A F (1996) Wound repair: overview and general considerations. *In* Clarke, R A F (ed) *The molecular and cellular biology of wound repair.* Plenum Press; New York, USA (2nd edition).
4. LEIBOLVITZ, S J; ROSS, R (1975) The role of the macrophage in wound repair: a study with hydrocortisone and antimacrophage serum. *American Journal of Pathology* 78: 71–100.
5. EAGLESTEIN, W H (1986) Wound healing and ageing. *Dermatologic Clinics* 4(3): 478–484.
6. OSHIMA, H; ROCHAT, A; KEDZIA, C; KOBAYASHI, K; BARRANDON, Y (2001) Morphogenesis and renewal of hair follicles from adult multipotent stem cells. *Cell* 104: 233–245.
7. DESAI, H (1997) Ageing and wounds. Part 2: healing in old age. *Journal of Wound Care* 6(4): 192–196.
8. KAWEL, K; POWELL, R J; SUMPIO, B E (1996) The pathology of diabetes mellitus: implications for surgeons. *Journal of the American College of Surgeons* 183(3): 271–289.
9. KNIGHTON, D R; HUNT, T K; SCHEUENSTUHL, H; HALLIDAYS, B J; WERB, Z; BANDA, M J (1983) Oxygen tension regulates the expression of angiogenesis factor by macrophages. *Science* 221: 1283–1285.
10. HUNT, T K; PAI, M P (1975) The effect of varying ambient oxygen tensions on wound metabolism and collagen synthesis. *Surgery, Gynaecology and Obstetrics* 135: 561–567.
11. PINCHROFSKY-DEVIN, G (1994) Nutritional wound healing. *Journal of Wound Care* 3(5): 231–234.
12. ÅGREN, M S; EAGLESTEIN, W H; FERGUSON, M W T; HARDING, K G; MOORE, K; SAARIALHO-KERE, U K; SCHULTZ, G S (2000). Causes and effects of the chronic inflammation in venous leg ulcers. *Acta Derm. Venereol.*. 210(Suppl): 3–17.
13. HANSSON, C; HOBORN, J; MÖLLER, A; SWANBECK, G (1995) The microbial flora in venous leg ulcers without clinical signs of infection. *Acta Derm. Venereol (Stockh)* 75: 24–30.

14. TRENGOVE, N; STACEY, M C; McGECHIE, D F; STINGEMORE, N F; MATA, S (1996) Qualitative bacteriology and leg ulcer healing. *Journal of Wound Care* 5(6): 277–280.
15. DALTREY, D C; RHODES, D; CHATTWOOD, J G (1981) Investigation into the microbial flora of healing and non-healing decubitus ulcers. *Journal of Clinical Pathology* 34: 701–705.
16. MADSEN, S M; WESTH, H; DANIELSEN, L; ROSDAHL, V T (1996) Bacterial colonisation and healing of venous ulcers. *APMIS* 104: 895–899.
17. HEPBURN, H H (1919) Delayed primary suture of wounds. *British Medical Journal* i: 181.
18. JACKSON, D M; LOWBURY, E J L; TOPLEY, E (1951) Chemotherapy of streptococcus infection of burns. *Lancet* 2: 705–711.
19. SCHRAIBMAN, I G (1990) The significance of β-haemolytic streptococci in chronic leg ulcers. *Annals of Royal College of Surgeons of England* 72: 123–124.
20. MOLAN, P C (1998) A brief review of honey as a clinical dressing. *Primary Intention* 6(4): 148–158.
21. MOLAN, P C (1999) The role of honey in the management of wounds. *Journal of Wound Care* 8(8): 415–418.
22. MOLAN, P C (1999) Why honey is effective as a medicine. Part 1. Its use in modern medicine. *Bee World* 80(2): 80–92.
23. MOLAN, P C (1992) The antibacterial activity of honey. 1. The nature of the antibacterial activity. *Bee World* 73(1): 5–28.
24. WILLIX, D J; MOLAN, P C; HARFOOT, C G (1992) A comparison of the sensitivity of wound infecting species of bacteria to the antibacterial activity of manuka honey and other honey. *Journal of Applied Bacteriology* 73: 388–394.
25. COOPER, R A; MOLAN, P C (1999) The use of honey as an antiseptic in managing *Pseduomonas* infection. *Journal of Wound Care* 8: 161–164.
26. COOPER, R A; MOLAN, P C; HARDING, K G (1999) Antibacterial activity of honey against strains of *Staphylococcus aureus* isolated from infected wounds. *Journal of Royal Society of Medicine* 92: 283–285.
27. COOPER, R A; WIGLEY, P; BURTON, N F (2000) Susceptibility of multiresistant strains of *Burkholderia cepacia* to honey. *Letters in Applied Microbiology* 31: 20–24.
28. DUNFORD, C; COOPER, R A; MOLAN, P C (2000) Using honey as a dressing for infected skin lesions. *Nursing Times (NT Plus)* 96(14): 7–9.
29. DUNFORD, C; COOPER, R A; MOLAN, P C; WHITE, R (2000) The use of honey in wound management. *Nursing Standard* 15(11): 63–68.
30. NATARAJAN, S; WILLIAMSON, D; GREY, J; HARDING, K G; COOPER, R A (2001) Healing of an MRSA colonised, hydroxyurea-induced leg ulcer with honey. *Journal of Dermatological Treatment* (in press).
31. SOFLER, A (1976) Chihuahuas and laetrile, chelation therapy, and honey from Boulder, Colorado. *Archives of Internal Medicine* 136: 865–866.
32. JONES, K P (2001) The role of honey in wound healing repair. *In* Munn, P A (ed.) *Honey and healing.* IBRA; Cardiff, UK; pp 35–36.

ROSE A COOPER

School of Applied Sciences, University of Wales Institute, Cardiff

The role of honey in wound healing and repair

KEN P JONES

The topical application of honey to wounds originated with ancient civilizations[1], persists in modern folk medicine, and has been rediscovered by modern professional physicians[2]. To date the evidence to support its efficacy in wound healing is largely anecdotal, but there are many claims that it reduces inflammation, debrides necrotic tissue, limits infections, sterilizes wounds, reduces oedema, sanitizes malodours, soothes local pain and promotes rapid angiogenesis, granulation and epithelialization[3,4]. Antibacterial activity of honey has been established in studies *in vitro*[5], but the mechanisms by which further therapeutic effects are achieved remain incompletely explained.

Wound healing is a complex process comprising both degenerative and reparative phases[6]. The tissue macrophages derived from peripheral blood monocytes are important agents in this process. They are intimately involved in the removal of damaged connective tissue and cell debris resulting from infection or injury, the killing and removal of pathogens, the formation of new blood vessels, the stimulation of fibroblast proliferation and resultant collagen synthesis gives rise to the subsequent remodelling of connective tissue. Macrophages, therefore, play a central role in regulating wound healing[7]. The primary response of macrophages to inflammatory stimuli following injury involves the release of powerful components aimed at stimulating the immune response, these are called cytokines. This is a very large group of compounds but amongst the most important of the macrophage derived cytokines is tumour necrosis factor alpha (TNF-α). Monocytes and macrophages are also involved in the production of reactive oxygen intermediates (ROIs) and hydrolytic enzymes, these are important in microbial killing. In addition they also produce growth factors and vasoactive agents which promote repair processes and aid recruitment of cells to the site of damage and the removal of dead or damaged cells.

TNF-α is a multifunctional cytokine which actively promotes inflammatory processes affecting almost every tissue and organ system. It potentiates the production of other cytokines thereby escalating levels of these cytokines[8] thus mediating actions other than those directly attributed to TNF-α. It is also known that TNF-α can prime and activate phagocytes[9] thus enhancing microbial removal. In macrophages and monocytes, phagocytosis is associated with an increase in oxygen consumption, oxidant generation and glucose catabolism via the hexose monophosphate shunt. This dramatic change in oxidative metabolism, usually referred to as the respiratory burst, can be induced by a variety of stimuli including phagocytosis[10].

The human monocytic cell line Mono Mac6 (MM6) was established in the late 1980s, offering many advantages over the then currently available U-937 and THP-1 cell lines[11]. This monocytic cell line has been proven to be extremely useful because to varying degree cells either constitutively or after stimulus express *in vitro* many of the properties manifested by their *in vivo* counterparts, mature peripheral blood monocytes and tissue macrophages.

We undertook a study to determine the effects of honey on the production of ROIs and TNF-α release in MM6 cells. It was felt that effects on these important pro-inflammatory responses may in part serve to explain the observed wound healing properties of honey. Activation of these cells by honey would suggest that honey in wounds may modulate repair mechanisms by up-regulating the activation state of macrophages and monocytes in the wound thus accelerating these systems. We used two varieties of New Zealand honey for the study as both had shown significant antimicrobial properties; these were manuka honey and a mixed pasture honey. As a control we used a sugar solution that contained the major sugars of honey in the appropriate concentrations. All of the honey samples were diluted before use in sterile pyrogen-free water. The honey was then incorporated into cell culture systems in which MM6 cells were either stimulated by a bacterial cell wall component, lipopolysaccharide, known to activate these cells, or were in a resting state.

The results of this investigation showed that honey at a concentration of 1% (w/v) can modulate the activation state of monocytic cells *in vitro*, but this does not affect the viability of these cells. This modulation can result in both inhibitory and stimulatory effects.

In respect of ROI production, manuka and pasture honey at 1% (w/v) concentration had a highly significant inhibitory effect on the production of reactive oxygen intermediates by activated MM6 cells. This effect was more pronounced with pasture honey than with manuka honey. The pasture honey was selected to be representative of honey generating relatively high levels of hydrogen peroxide[3]. It is possible that when MM6 cells were preincubated with this diluted honey, a negative feedback on the production of reactive oxygen intermediate species resulted from the honey-derived hydrogen peroxide. In undiluted honeys the concentration of hydrogen peroxide is usually low, but on dilution glucose oxidase derived from bees is activated and generates gluconic acid and hydrogen peroxide from glucose and oxygen. The hydrogen peroxide is thought to inhibit bacteria[5]. Manuka honey produces smaller quantities of hydrogen peroxide and this, in part, could explain the differences seen between the two. No such effect was observed with the artificial honey

A marked effect on spontaneous release of TNF-α from resting MM6 cells was seen with 1% (w/v) manuka and pasture honey. Both these honeys induced significant production of TNF-α from resting MM6 cells, whereas the artificial honey did not. This would suggest that a component or components within these natural honeys may directly stimulate these cells. Interestingly neither honey influenced TNF-α release in stimulated cells, suggesting a mechanism other than that induced by lipopolysaccharide.

The components in honey responsible for the modulation of MM6 responses seen in this study have not yet been elucidated. The effect of honey on cell lines has not yet been extensively studied. Honey at lower concentrations than those used in this study has been shown to have mitogenic activity on human B- and T-lymphocytes and phagocytes[13], and a protein fractionated from royal jelly has been demonstrated to stimulate U-937 human myeloid cell line[14]. Proteins present in honey will invariably be highly glycosylated because of the high sugar content, glycosylated proteins have been shown to cause significant activation of a number of cell types[15].

The anecdotal evidence that honey aids wound healing may in part be due to the stimulatory effects of glycosylated honey proteins or as yet unidentified components on macrophages. These cells are known to be important in wound healing and tissue repair[16]. The importance of TNF-α in the healing process has been stressed by a number of authors[17,18]. The reduction in ROIs seen in the presence of honey may serve to limit tissue damage by activated macrophages during the healing process. Leakage of these components from activated cells is responsible for much of the tissue damage associated with inflammation. Thus, honey may aid in the healing process by both activating cells important in this mechanism and also by limiting the production of potentially damaging components normally associated with these cells when activated.

REFERENCES

1. FORREST, R D (1982) Early history of wound treatment. *Journal of the Royal Society of Medicine* 75: 198–205.
2. ZUMLA, A; LULAT, A (1989) Honey — a remedy re-discovered. *Journal of the Royal Society of Medicine* 82: 384–385.
3. MOLAN, P C (1998) A brief review of honey as a clinical dressing. *Primary Intention* 6(4): 148–58.
4. MOLAN, P C (1999) The role of honey in the management of wounds. *Journal of Wound Care* 8(8): 415–418.
5. MOLAN, P C (1992) The antibacterial activity of honey. 1. The nature of the antibacterial activity. *Bee World* 73(1): 5–28.
6. CLARKE, R A F (1996) Wound repair. In Clarke, R A F (ed) *The molecular and cellular biology of wound repair.* Plenum Press; New York, USA; pp 3–50 (2nd edition).
7. RICHENS, D W H (1996) Macrophage involvement in wound repair, remodelling and fibrosis. In Clarke, R A F (ed) *The molecular and cellular biology of wound repair.* Plenum Press; New York, USA; pp 95–141 (2nd edition).
8. AGGARWAL, B B; VILECK, J (1992) *Tumor necrosis factors: structure, function and mechanisms of action.* Marcel Dekker; New York, USA.
9. MOORE, F D JR; SOCHER, S H; DAVIS, C (1991) Tumor necrosis factor and endotoxin can cause neutrophil activation through separate pathways. *Arch Surg.* 126(1): 70–73.
10. FELS, A; COHN, Z (1986) The alveolar macrophage. *Journal of Applied Physiology* 60(2): 353–369.
11. ZIEGLER-HEITBROCK, H W; SCHRAUCT, W; STRÖBEL, M; STERNSDORF, T; WEBER, C; AEPFELBACHER, A; EHLERS, M; SCHÜTT, C; HASS, J (1994) Distinct patterns of differentiation induced in the monocytic cell line Monomac6. *Journal of Leukocyte Biology* 55: 73–80.
12. ALLEN, R; MEAD, M; KELLY, J (1986) Phagocyte oxygenation activity measured by chemiluminescence and chemilumingenic probing. *CRC Handbook of Methods for Oxygen Radical Research*; pp 343–350.
13. ABUHARFEIL, N; ALORAN, R; ABOSHEHADA, M (1999) The effect of bee honey on the proliferative activity of human B and T-lymphocytes and the activity of phagocytes. *Food and Agricultural Immunology* 11(2): 169–177.
14. WATANABE, K; SHINMOTO, H; KOBORI, M; TSUSHIDA, T; SHINOHARA, K; KANAEDA, J; YONEKURA, M (1998) Stimulation of cell growth in the U-937 human myeloid cell line by honey royal jelly protein. *Cytotechnology* 26: 23–27.
15. BROWNLEE, M (1995) Advanced protein glycosolation diabetes and aging. *Annual Review of Medicine* 46: 223–34.
16. DYSON, M; YOUNG, S R; PENDLE, C L; WEBSTER, D F; LANG, S M (1988) Comparison of the effects of moist and dry conditions on dermal repair. *Journal of Investigative Dermatology* 9: 435–39.
17. MOORE, K; THOMAS, A; HARDING, K G (1997) Iodine released from the wound dressing Iodosorb modulates the secretion of cytokines by human macrophages responding to lipopolysaccharide. *International Journal of Biochemical Cell Biolology* 29: 163–71.

KEN P JONES
School of Applied Sciences, University of Wales Institute, Cardiff.

Stingless bee honey and the treatment of cataracts

PATRICIA VIT

HUMAN CATARACTS

At least 50 million people suffer from cataract-related visual impairments, with 17 million being severely disabled. In the UK, cataracts are one of the four main causes of blindness. Half of the blindness in the world is due to cataracts and this represents some 13 million people[9] of which more than 90% are in developing countries[35]. Senile and diabetic cataracts are of epidemiological interest in human populations.

The lens of the human eye has no blood vessels, is transparent and biconvex, with aqueous humour on the anterior face and vitreous humour on the posterior and more convex face. A cataract is formed when the ocular lens becomes clouded or opaque. Loss of lens transparency may result from a variety of reasons causing light scattering due to microstructural stress within the lens. Proteins become denatured and the water content increases in cataract lens fibres[5].

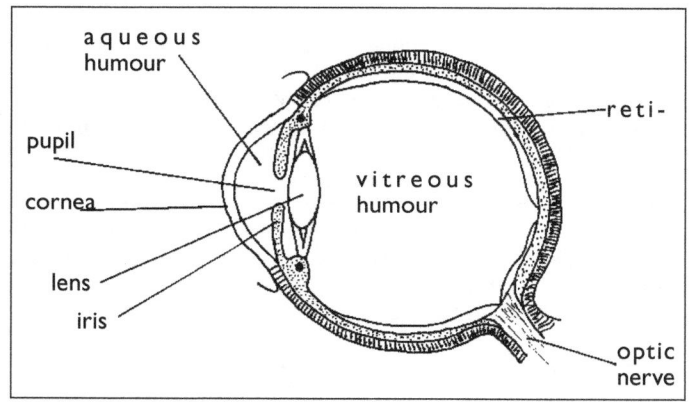

Cross-section through the human eye.

MEDICAL TREATMENT

When a cataract is severe enough to impair vision, the lens is removed surgically with or without intraocular lens implantation[14,34]. However, vision impairment often develops as a postoperative complication caused by the proliferation of epithelial cells and macrophages on the posterior capsule[15].

Medical therapies may be able to prevent, retard or reverse lens opacity[4]. A delay of cataract onset by 10 years would reduce by 45% the number of cataract operations[17]. The rationale for anticataract agents is based on the type of cataract, targeting specific cataract-inducing mechanisms. Protection is afforded by the lens in the form of antioxidant or osmotic balance capacity[8,13,14]. The use of different anticataract agents is a common practice although their action on cataracts has not been supported properly by clinical trials[12,36].

HONEY INSTILLATIONS AND FLAVONOIDS

Topical therapy is the preferred method of treatment. Both topical and systemic drugs require lipid solubility for penetration[4], and water solubility for humoral diffusion and concentration. To gain access to the lens, the active agent of the honey should have lipid and water solubility to cross the cornea[6,20] and the ability to

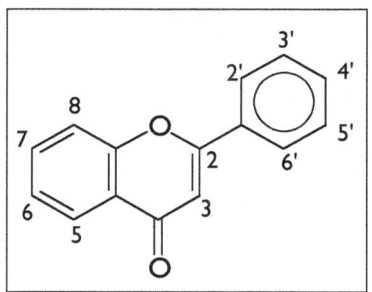

Structural skeleton of a flavonoid.

concentrate in the aqueous humour after instillations. Flavonoids present in stingless bee honey[33] could meet these chemical requirements.

Flavonoids are found in honey as residual secondary plant metabolites. They have been studied as potential botanical and geographical markers for characterizing honey sources[1,10,23,26,27,28], and also to explain the antibacterial properties of honey[3]. In eye research, flavonoids have been reported as anticataract agents in vivo[30] and in vitro[21,25,29] because of their osmotic protection as inhibitors of aldose reductase. However, flavonoids have not been previously explored in connection with the putative anticataract attributes of honey instillations.

MELIPONICULTURE AND FOLK TRADITIONS

Stingless bee honey is traditionally considered to be more powerful than honey bee honey for use as a 'natural' medicine for treating common diseases. For example, in some regions, particular stingless bee species are thought to produce honey that stimulates human fertility, and in others honey is given to help during childbirth.

The most unexpected and fascinating application is the traditional use of stingless-bee honey as eye-drops for cataract treatment. This is an ancient Amerindian tradition mentioned in the Mayan Pharmacopea. Commercial honey eye-drops are produced in several countries and are reputed to cure cataracts and other eye diseases: e.g. honeys from *Melipona favosa favosa* ('erica') and *Trigona angustula angustula* ('angelita') are used in Venezuela; *M. beecheii* and *Scaptotrigona mexicana* in Mexico; and *T. a. angustula* ('jataí') in Brazil. In Venezuela, the basic treatment is undiluted honey. Preferences for different honeys produced by different species of stingless bee occur in different countries, often based on the abundance of the stingless bee species in a location. Additions of plant extracts have also been observed, mainly of the Solanaceae (e.g. *Physalis peruviana*) and Asteraceae (e.g. *Cineraria maritima*) families.

EXPERIMENTAL APPROACH

Honey, flavonoids and cataracts

The presence of phenolic compounds is a characteristic feature of plant tissues, and flavonoids are the largest group of these phenolics. These secondary plant metabolites are also present in the phenolic extracts of plant-derived products such as honey.

Although bee products are used to treat eye diseases, their effects on cataracts are not supported by solid data. However, there is some published research. Golichev[11] recommended vitamin intake and diluted honey to treat cortical and incipient senile cataracts after a study with 108 patients in Russia. Visual acuity was maintained in 80% of 2492 patients presenting incipient cataracts treated with honey, royal jelly and propolis ophthalmic solutions in Rumania[22]. In neotropical countries, stingless bee honeys from *M. beecheii*, *M. favosa favosa* and *T. angustula angustula* have putative properties to cure or delay the process of senile cataracts by use of diluted and direct instillations in the eye[32]. The osmotic stress theory for causing cataracts provided Kinoshita[16] with the rationale for the use of aldose reductase inhibitors (ARI) to prevent osmotic swelling caused by intracellular polyol accumulation in sugar cataracts. Potent synthetic ARI are the strongest potential anticataract agents tested to date[14]. In 1976 Varma[29] presented evidence of a new biological activity of flavonoids, relating these plant compounds with anticataract effects.

The role of flavonoids in preventing cataracts has been associated with their inhibitory activity of lens aldose reductase. In a classic enzymatic study where 44 flavonoids were screened as ARI, apigenin was the strongest inhibitor in the group of di- and trihydroxyflavones[29]. However, in another study, the aldose reductase inhibitory activity was low for apigenin and isorhamnetin, but high for luteolin[25]. Luteolin content was greater in *Melipona* than in *A. mellifera* phenolic extracts of Venezuelan honeys[33]. In another report, it was indicated that monoglycosides have a higher aldose reductase activity than the corresponding aglycone, except for luteolin[21]. Methylated flavonoids were more effective than non-methylated flavonoids in inhibiting sorbitol formation in sugar cataracts[7].

The swelling of lens fibres under hyperglycaemic stress is associated with the increase of intracellular sorbitol. However, despite the high levels of intracellular sorbitol, the osmotic stress was controlled to some degree in lenses treated with myoinositol or antioxidants[2], suggesting that probably the loss of membrane integrity is not due to osmotic stress alone, but also to alteration of membrane components[19]. This dual osmotic and oxidative protection of membrane integrity was inferred from similar losses of GSH in diabetic and oxidative cataracts[18]. Vitamin C and flavonoids also gave simultaneous protection of the lens against the damaging effects of oxyradicals and polyols[31].

Lens culture and *in vivo* models

Three opacity models were explored by digital image analysis of cultured sheep lenses:

Chapter six: Meliponinae honey and cataracts

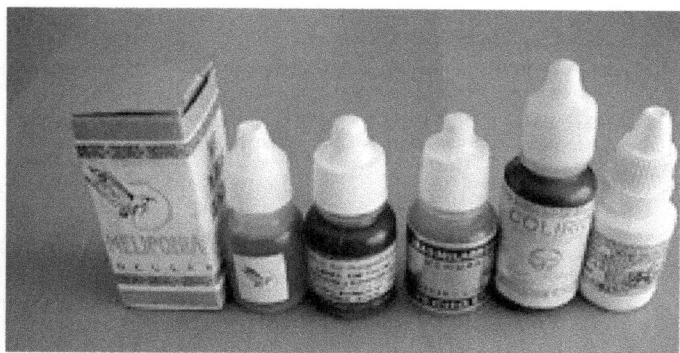

Commercially available stingless bee honey eye-drops.

- Graded hypotonicity (i.e. varying the osmotic pressure).
- Hypocalcaemic regime (i.e. reducing the level of calcium).
- Hyperglycaemic regime (i.e. increasing the level of sugar).

The time course of average grey level (polar view) response was measured over a 24-h period. Departures of grey level from control lenses represent loss of transparency due to increased light scatter and may be caused/produced by a multifactorial process (swelling, calcium binding, glycation of proteins, oxidation, ionic imbalance) that remained undetermined in the present work. From 20 commercial flavonoids that might be present in stingless bee honey, four luteolin derivatives reduced the lens opacity caused by hypotonic stress. The control of loss of transparency by luteolin tetramethylether varied locally according to the modelling stress imposed:

- In the hyperglycaemic regime, it was partial and localized in a thin anterior equatorial ring.
- In the other two models it was localized in the posterior cap of approximately one third of the polar axis, it was partial in the 45% hypotonic media and complete in the hypocalcaemic regime.
- Luteolin had a protective effect if applied during the control phase of both regimes.

These results suggest that other mechanisms different from control of polyol accumulation might be implicated in the flavonoid ability to control lens opacity.

The effect of stingless bee honey eye-drops was tested in two *in vivo* models, based on diabetic cataract[16] and selenite cataract[24]. However, the high variability in the response did not lead to conclusive results. A group of rats presented delayed cataract in the eye treated with a daily drop of honey over two weeks after exposure to the cataract-inducing agent. Extended *in vivo* experiments are needed.

FUTURE WORK

Some derivatives of the luteolin family reduced the degree of opacity in cultured lenses under hypotonic stress, hypocalcaemic and hyperglycaemic regimes. Until their mechanisms of action become understood, it would be wise to bear in mind that other factors are possibly involved. Specific efforts should be addressed to answer questions at the membrane, crystalline and enzymatic level, to start to unravel the mechanisms involved. The role of the capsule should also be explored, looking at the process of cataract formation and recovery, its physicochemical response towards cataract-inducing regimes and inhibition or regression induced by flavonoids, as well as the implications of induced epithelial attachment-detachment.

This preliminary study of experimental cataract formation needs fundamental biochemical, morphological and histological support; not only to complete the descriptive framework of the intact lens but also to provide a basis for approaching the major mechanisms involved and to explore what are the targets of the flavonoids that might be involved with the protection of lens transparency.

The degree of lens clouding is the obvious variable to describe the visual impairment caused by cataracts, but it is a sequence of metabolic events that result in the light scatter in its final stage. For that reason, indicators of defined metabolic routes preceding the lens clouding are necessary to detect what the mechanisms involved are and to explain how they may interact. An integral system should embrace optimised indicators having high correlation with the degree of clouding generated in each cataract-inducing model, measured as grey level in digital images. It will be very profitable to correlate both geometric and biochemical indicators with the measurement of lens transparency.

If the lens cells cannot control their volume, the lens swells and loses transparency. Therefore increases in lens volume could be correlated with the degree of opacity. Added to the physical changes, sorbitol content or protein glycation would be good indicators for the hyperglycaemic regime and free calcium for the hypocalcaemic regime. Although water content seems the most obvious measurement for the graded hypotonicity, other biochemical parameters should be explored for their ability to predict, not only the degree of opacity, but also changes preceding it.

Finally, the animal model and the epidemiological studies will permit an evaluation of what tradition says about the anticataract properties of stingless bee honey but was never measured, namely; whether the human cataract is delayed or prevented by this treatment.

REFERENCES

1. AMIOT, M J; AUBERT, S; GONNET, M; TACCHINI, M (1989) Les composés phénoliques des miels: étude préliminaire sur l'identification et la quantification par familles. *Apidologie* 20(2): 115–125.
2. BEYER-MEARS, A; BUCCI, F A; DEL VAL, M; CRUZ, E (1989) Dietary myoinositol effect on sugar cataractogenesis. *Pharmacology* 39(1): 59–68.
3. BOGDANOV, S (1984) Characterisation of antibacterial substances in honey. *Lebensmittel Wissenschaft Technologie* 17(2): 74–76.
4. BRON, A J; BROWN, N A P; SPARROW, J M; SHUN SHIN, G A (1987) Medical treatment of cataract. *Eye* 1(5): 542–550.
5. BROWN, N A P; BRON, A J (1985) Medical therapy in the prevention of cataract. *Transactions of the Ophthalmological Society of the United Kingdom* 104(7): 748–754.
6. CHANALET, L; LAPALUS, P (1994) Drugs designed to maintain the transparency of the ocular lens. *Fundamental & Clinical Pharmacology* 8(4): 322–341.
7. CHIOU, G C Y; STOLOWICH, N J; ZHENG, Y Q; SHEN, Z F; ZHU, M; MIN, Z D (1992) Effects of some natural products on sugar cataract studied with nuclear magnetic resonance spectroscopy. *Journal of Ocular Pharmacology* 8(2): 115–120.
8. DE SANTIS, L (1986) New horizons in the medical therapy of cataract:: aldose reductase inhibitors and other agents. *Pharmacy International* 7(1): 17–20.
9. DOUTHWAITE, W A (1993) Introduction. *In* Douthwaite, W A; Hurst, M A (eds) *Cataract: detection, measurement and management in optometric practice*. Butterworth-Heinemann; Oxford, UK; pp. 1–3.
10. FERRERES, F; GARCÍA VIGUERA, C; TOMÁS-LORENTE, F; TOMÁS-BARBERÁN, F A (1993) Hesperetin: a marker of the floral origin of *Citrus* honeys. *Journal of the Science of Food and Agriculture* 61(1): 121–123.
11. GOLICHEV, V N (1990) Honey in conservative therapy of senile cataract. *Vestnik Oftalmologii* 6: 59–62.
12. HARDING, J J (1991) *Cataract: biochemistry, epidemiology and pharmacology*. Chapman & Hall; London, UK; 333 pp.
13. HARDING, J J (1992) Pharmacological treatment strategies in age-related cataracts. *Drugs & Aging* 2(4): 287–300.
14. KADOR, P F (1983) Overview of the current attempts toward the medical treatment of cataract. *Ophthalmology* 90(4): 352–364.
15. KAPPELHOF, J P; VRENSEN, F J M (1992) Pathology of after-cataract. *Acta Ophthalmologica* 205(s): 13–24.
16. KINOSHITA, J H (1974) Mechanisms initiating cataract formation. *Investigative Ophthalmology* 13(10): 713–724.
17. KUPFER, C (1984) The conquest of cataract: a global challenge. Bowman Lecture. *Transactions of the Ophthalmological Society of the United Kingdom* 104(1): 1–10.
18. MÅRTENSSON, J; MEISTER, A (1991) Glutathione deficiency decreases tissue ascorbate levels in newborn rats: ascorbate spares glutathione and protects. *Proceedings of the National Academy of Sciences of the United States of America* 8(11): 4656–4560.
19. MITTON, K P; PAW, D; DZIALOSYNSKI, T; XIONG, H; SANFORD, S E; TREVITHICK, J R (1993) Modelling cortical cataractogenesis 13. Early effects on lens ATP/ADP and glutathione in the streptozotocin rat model of the diabetic cataract. *Experimental Eye Research* 56(2): 187–198.
20. O'CONNOR DAVIES, P H; HOPKINS, G A; PEARSON, R M (1989) *The actions and uses of ophthalmic drugs*. Butterworths; London, UK; 248 pp (3rd edition).
21. OKUDA, J; MIWA, I; INAGAKI, K; HORIE, T; NAKAYAMA, M (1982) Inhibition of aldose reductases from rat and bovine lenses by flavonoids. *Biochemical Pharmacology* 31: 3807–3822.
22. POPESCU, M P; POPESCU, D A (1993) Use of the bee products in the treatment of incipient lens opacifications. *Programme and Abstracts of Reports XXXIII International Congress of Apiculture*. Apimondia; Beijing, China; p. 134.
23. SABATIER, S; AMIOT, M J; TACCHINI, M; AUBERT, S (1992) Identification of flavonoids in sunflower honey. *Journal of Food Science* 57(3): 773–774, 777.
24. SHEARER, T R; DAVID, L L; ANDERSON, R S; AZUMA, M (1992) Review of selenite cataract. *Current Eye Research* 11(4): 357–369.
25. SHIMIZU, M; ITO, T; TERASHIMA, S; HAYASHI, T; ARISAWA, M; MORITA, N; KUROKAWA, S; ITO, K; HASHIMOTO, Y (1984) Inhibition of lens aldose reductase by flavonoids. *Phytochemistry* 23: 1885–1888.
26. SOLER, C; GIL, M; GARCÍA-VIGUERA, C; TOMÁS-BARBERÁN, F A (1995) Flavonoid patterns of French honeys with different floral origin. *Apidologie* 26(1): 53–60.
27. TOMÁS-BARBERÁN, F A; FERRERES, F; BLÁZQUEZ, M A; GARCÍAVIGUERA, C; TOMÁS-LORENTE, F (1993) High-performance liquid chromatography of honey flavonoids. *Journal of Chromatography* 634: 41–46.
28. TOMÁS-BARBERÁN, F A; FERRERES, F; GARCÍA-VIGUERA, C; TOMÁS-LORENTE, F (1993) Flavonoids in honey of different geographical origin. *Zeitschrift für Lebensmittel-Untersuchung und-Forschung* 196(1): 38–44.
29. VARMA, S D; KINOSHITA, J H (1976) Inhibition of lens aldose reductase by flavonoids -their possible role in the prevention of diabetic cataracts. *Biochemical Pharmacology* 25: 2505–2513.
30. VARMA, S D; MIZUNO, A; KINOSHITA, J H (1977) Diabetic cataracts and flavonoids. *Science* 195(4274): 205–206.
31. VARMA, S D; RAMACHANDRAN, S; DEVAMANOHARAN, P S; HENEIN, M (1992) Simultaneous prevention of lens against the damaging effects of oxyradicals and polyols by vitamin C and flavonoids. Abstract. *Investigative Ophthalmology & Visual Science* 33(4): 866.

PATRICIA VIT

Facultad de Farmacia, Universidad de los Andes, Mérida, Venezuala

The treatment of burns and other wounds with honey

Theo Postmes

BURNS AND FIRST AID

Imagine you are camping and your daughter burns her hand with hot water — what are you going to do? Fortunately, most people know the first rule for treating burns, which says: cool with water for at least 10 minutes. But what should you do next? If you have an English first aid book, then you can read that you have to treat burns and scalds, caused by steam or hot liquids, in exactly the same way. A brief summary of the recommendations follow[1]:

1. Douse the burn with copious amounts of cold liquid for 10 minutes or more.
2. Gently remove any watches, jewellery, belts, shoes, or smouldering/burned clothing, but **not** if the clothing is sticking to the burn.
3. Cover the injury with a sterile burns sheet if possible, or improvise with clean, non-fluffy material, until seen by a doctor or nurse. DO NOT use adhesive dressings or strapping.
4. DO NOT touch or otherwise interfere with the burned area.
5. DO NOT apply fat, ointments or lotions to the injury.
6. DO NOT burst any blisters.
7. For severe burns and scalds, seek medical assistance as soon as possible. Check airway, breathing and pulse. All deep burns of any size must receive hospital attention[2].

Burns and scalds are the same all over the world, but the first aid advice may depend on what country you are in. For example, the minimum time recommended for cooling with water is: 5 minutes in The Netherlands, Belgium, France and Chile; 10 minutes in the UK, Ireland, Spain, USA and Australia; 15 minutes in Canada; and 30 minutes in Venezuela.

MAJOR AND MINOR BURNS

Deep burns require special attention — what are deep burns? The answer is given in figure 1. When all layers of the skin are burned you have a deep (full thickness) burn, a so-called 'third degree' burn. Since the nerves are damaged you don't feel pain. On the other hand, a partial-thickness burn ('second degree') may be very painful. An infection in the wound may easily turn it into a third-degree burn. Mild sunburn is usually gone after one day — a superficial ('first degree') burn — however, it is more serious if you have blisters and are as red as a lobster.

Any size of full-thickness burn requires medical attention. With an indoor fire toxic gases are inhaled and these may lead to respiratory and circulatory problems. The patient may be in shock and in need of acute burn management. Loss of water, salt and protein after shock require a resuscitation procedure. Highly specialized burns units have a computer system, *a patient-simulator*, which is able to calculate the right infusion of liquid. To optimize this complex process one has to deal with 190 equations and about 400 constants and variables[3].

The definition of *minor burns* is usually linked to the total body surface area (TBSA) affected. Small burns are easy to treat. Up to 30% of TBSA can be treated by a GP or a local hospital. The 'rules of nine' are used to calculate the extent of the burn as a percentage of the TBSA:

- An arm is always 9% of TBSA whether you are 1, 5 or 70 years old.
- The head is also 9%.
- Front and back of the chest are each 18% (2×9).
- Front and back of legs are each 9% (each whole leg being 18%).
- Crotch: 1%.

In short, a child 5 years of age with a second-degree burn of 7×7 cm on the inner side of her arm has a TBSA of less than 2%. After cooling (see above) you can immediately cover the wound with a sterile gauze with honey on top. A paper tissue as a second layer may prevent leakage of the sticky honey. Most minor burns and scalds will heal within two or three weeks.

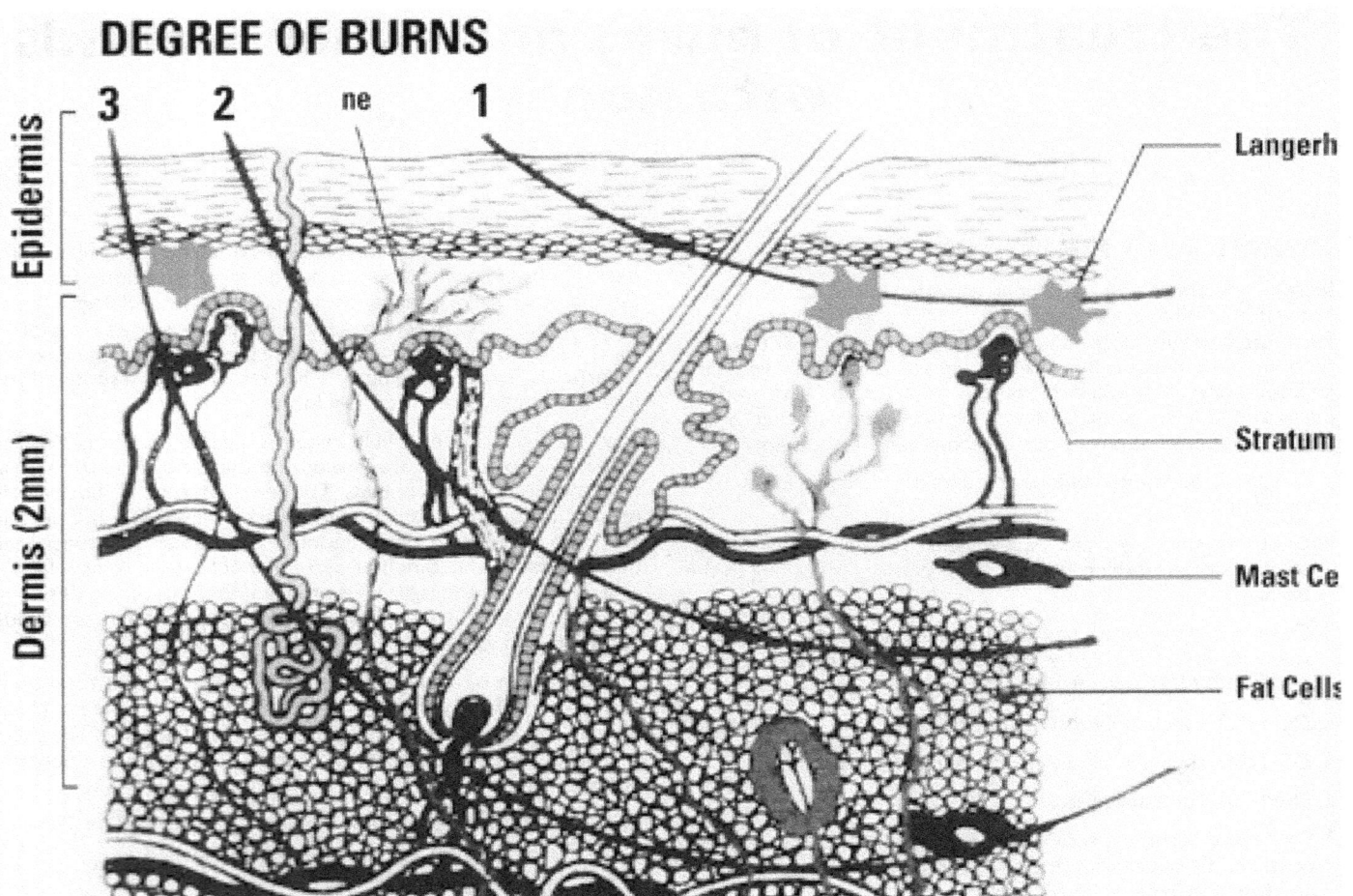

FIG. 1. Different types of burn. In first-degree burns (1) only the surface of the skin, the epidermis, is damaged. Characteristics are redness, mild pain and swelling. After a deep second-degree burn (2) the skin looks pale and the nerve endings (ne) are damaged. Living epithelial cells are frequently found in the remains of hair roots, sebaceous glands and sweat glands. The patient feels pain, like being pricked with a pin. General characteristics are blisters, raw red skin, swelling and extreme pain. After third-degree burns (3) the blood vessels and nerves are so badly damaged that all feeling is lost and the skin is dead. Re-epithelialization can only start from the edges of the wound. Skin grafts are often required. Characteristics are no pain, the skin may appear pale or waxy, and sometimes has a charred appearance.

EPIDEMIOLOGY

In the UK a fair estimate of the annual incidence of burns is about 4.7 per 1000 of the population. About 80% of all burns occur at home and young children are especially at risk[3]. In the Netherlands the overall incidence figure is 775 per 100 000 children aged 0–4 years old and only 133 per 100 000 people in the 55+ age group[4]. Before entering school one child in 130 is likely to have been admitted to hospital as a consequence of sustaining a burn or a scald. About 75% of all thermal injuries could have been prevented. Arms and/or hands are the parts of the body that are most frequently affected and are responsible for 65% of all burns.

In the population of Maastricht of the very young, between one and four years, only 3% are referred to a special burns unit; 31.2% are treated in a local hospital. The majority of all burns (65.8%) are seen by a GP[5]. Statistics of the true incidence of injury, death or disability in many countries such as India, Indonesia and China are mostly limited to a few big cities, and data for people living in the country are lacking.

In short: the statistics show that the majority of burns can be classified as minor thermal injuries.

EXPERIMENTAL BURNS

Since one aspect of the wound-healing properties of honey is based on the stimulation of lymph drainage by the water-bearing potential of the various sugars in the honey solution, white sugar (sucrose) might be an alternative for honey. So, shouldn't we use sugar to treat burns instead of honey? Actually granulated sugar has been tested many times and Drouet[5] and Keith et al.[6] have presented interesting reviews of various clinical trials.

Both white sugar and honey have something in common, however, honey is far more complex. Honey contains trace elements (copper, zinc, iodine, manganese), vitamins (B_1 (thiamine), B_2 complex and C), a great number of flavonoids (antioxidants), 13 different disaccharides, 15 trisaccharides and higher sugars up to 1.5%, proline (an amino acid which is a precursor of collagen), aroma constituents, and straight-chain fatty acids, etc. Many kinds of honey have a high antibacterial activity due to the presence of hydrogen peroxide. Incidentally, the wound fluid rapidly dilutes undiluted honey put on a wound. Several studies have shown that hydrogen peroxide is generated by glucose oxidase, an enzyme. The activity of this enzyme is optimal in diluted honey up to a concentration of 30%[7,8,9].

SILVER SULFADIAZINE, SUGAR AND HONEY

Comparative studies show that the skin of the pig, which has relatively few hair follicles, best matches that of a human. The pig's

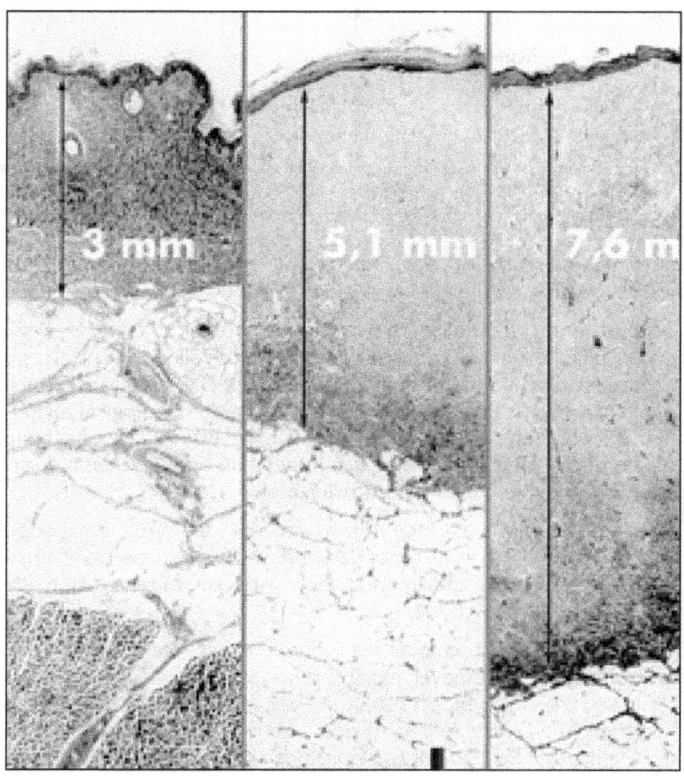

FIG. 2. Pig skin. (a) Normal pig's skin with subcutaneous fat (under arrow), original enlargement ¥ 12.5; PAP stain. **(b)** Pig 137: honey side, day 28, illustrates that the epidermis is intact, indicating full epithelialization. Enlargement and staining as in (a). **(c)** Pig 137: sugar side, day 28, the dermis is markedly thicker than in (b). Enlargement and colouring as in (a).

TABLE 1. The Yorkshire pig pilot study with experimental deep second-degree burns treated with honey, silver sulfadiazine (SSD) or sugar paste (artificial honey). All skin thickness data are particularly related to the middle part of the wound.

Pig no.	Treatment	100% Epithelialization (days)	Dermis[1] after: 14	21	28	35	42 days
120	honey	21–28[2]	1.7	3.3	2.7	2.9	3.0
	SSD	28–35[2]	1.0	1.1	2.7	3.3	2.8
64	honey	21	3.3	1.5	2.0	2.0	1.7
	honey	21	2.5	2.3	1.8	1.5	1.7
137	Sugar	21	1.8	3.5	2.7	2.3	2.2
	honey	21	1.3	2.5	1.5	1.3	2.4

[1] The thickness of the skin (epidermis and dermis) in the middle of the wound is calculated in relation to normal skin, which is 3–4 mm thick in most places.
[2] On day 21, the wound is almost closed and epithelialization is nearly 100%. The next measurement is taken on day 28, so the 100% point lies between day 21 and 28.

physiology also shows clear similarities, and this is important for the study of systemic effects during severe burns.

Second- and third-degree burns can be treated adequately with silver sulfadiazine (SSD), sugar or honey in the clinic. SSD is a topical cream that is very effective against bacterial infections, which explains why it is used in most burns units. As a histological examination in human patients is not possible for ethical reasons, tests of the effectiveness of SSD *versus* honey and honey *versus* a sugar solution have been carried out using pigs.

The experiments described below were carried out according to Hoekstra *et al.*[11] and in accordance with Dutch Law on Animal Experimentation. Experimental second-degree burns were made on pigs under anaesthesia.

It is vitally important that all the wounds are as similar as possible. Of course, they are never exactly the same because the skin varies in thickness and blood supply. A way around this problem is to compare one on the left-hand side with one at the same place on the right side. Each week (on post-burn days 7, 14, 21, 28, 35 and 42) biopsies were taken symmetrically from wounds on the left and right flanks. Biopsies included the wound bed as well as the healthy skin of the wound margins. Tissue fixing and staining were as described previously[11]. The main results of the pilot study are shown in figure 2 and in table 1 (for more details see Postmes[10]).

The results of the pilot study show above all that all the wounds treated with honey or sugar healed at least one week earlier than with SSD. Macroscopically it is almost impossible to assess the degree of epithelialization due to the presence of the crust. By definition, the wound is considered 'closed and healed' if the epidermis is found microscopically uninterrupted. Normally, repair of the epidermis is due to the outgrowth of epithelial cells at the edge of the wound. However, hair follicle cells, which still possess vital epithelial cells, are also included in the process of re-epithelialization. With SSD cream many of the epithelial cells do not survive and others are inhibited by the uptake of SSD. In sugar- and in SSD-treated burns the deeper layers of skin showed an ongoing inflammation of small blood vessels and hair follicles. Chronic inflammations were even found after the wound was fully closed. Micro-inflammatory loci are almost absent in the honey-treated burns.

The actual thickness of the skin against time is a different story. On the one hand we see for instance on day 28 a structure which is not normal skin (see fig. 2), but rather a repair in the form of a scar. At this stage or later wound contraction may occur with SSD but not with honey. Wound contractions, caused by some persistent deep dermal inflammations, may often invalidate the patient. On the other hand figures 2b and c show microscopically a scar and a neodermis, which is far thicker than the dermis of the healthy skin next to the injured area. In this pilot study, the impression gained was that the dermis of wounds treated with sugar was generally thicker than in those treated with honey. Only day 42 is an exception.

Burns treated with honey show very low inflammatory reactions in contrast to the SSD-treated burns. The honey-treated burns enter their end phase within six weeks, which is unique and not seen with any other wound dressing[12].

In short: the pig study showed that the number of nursing days can be reduced by 25%. The experiments showed honey to be superior to SSD, the 'golden standard' of today. The results suggest also that we ought to change the first aid protocol for minor burns.

CLINICAL STUDIES

Experimental studies may show us how we might treat burns in the best way. However, it is clinical trials that tell us if our extrapolations were right. Whenever damage to tissue occurs there is always a risk of infection, fluid loss and wound shock. Although the efficacy of honey in preventing infection has been reported many times, as yet no evidence is available from comparative, randomized studies. These are studies planned in advance in which the selection process of subjects is set up in a deliberately random way to enhance the statistical validity. An ideal way to achieve really sound data is through a double-blind study. This means that neither the patients nor the attending physician know whether the patient is being treated with a placebo or the active substance. In the treatment of burns, a double-blind trial with honey is simply out of the question.

What is possible is a randomized, comparative study with honey on the one side and SSD on the other (table 2). The data in table 2 show clearly that honey is more effective than SSD. The antibacterial action of SSD is achieved by silver ions, which in fact are not completely harmless[14,15]. After seven days of honey therapy, 91% of the wounds were free of bacteria as compared with 7% in the control group. What is possibly even more important is that less pain and less scarring were found in the honey group than in the comparable SSD group.

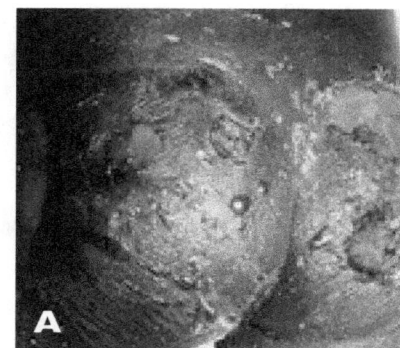
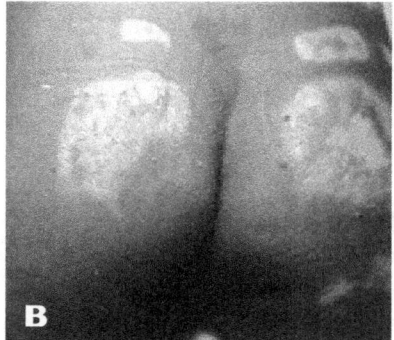

An Indian patient with blisters (first-degree burn) and second-degree burns (a).

The same patient after eight days of treatment with honey (b). The wound is clean and healing nicely. The skin's colour has not yet returned to normal, but, according to Subrahmanyam, pigmentation returns at a later stage.

Many patients with thermal injuries were treated with honey by Professor Subrahmanyam in his clinic in Solapur (India). In a very large comparative randomized study, honey was used for minor burns or so-called partial-thickness burns. Over a six-year period, 450 patients (< 40% TBSA) were treated with honey and the results were compared to those obtained in 450 patients treated by conventional methods in the same period[16]. Most wounds treated with honey healed earlier than those treated conventionally (8.8

Treatment	Surface area of burn*	End infection	100% healing
Silver sulfadiazine ($n = 52$)	5–40%	7 days (7%)	15 days (10%)
Honey ($n = 52$)	5–40%	7 days (91%)	15 days (87%)

TABLE 2. A summary of the treatment results. For further details on age, sex and type of burn see Subrahmanyam[13].

days versus 13.5 days). Further, residual scars occurred far less in the honey treated patients than those treated conventionally (6.2% versus 19.7%).

According to Efem[17], inadequacies and side effects often seen in wound treatment do not apply to a honey dressing because its main properties are: cleansing, absorption of oedemal fluids, antimicrobial activity, deodorization, promotion of granulation tissue formation, epithelization, and improvement of nutrition. A notable feature is also the chemical debridement action of honey and its absorption by the wound. In practice, a gauze with a honey layer on top remains moist and adheres little, if at all, to the wound surface. And most important of all, honey has never been reported to be toxic.

In conclusion, burns that are treated with honey heal more rapidly and effectively in a patient-friendly way, without infection complications, and with little pain and relatively little scarring. Honey treatment of burns is certainly cost effective because it shortens the duration of treatment by c. 25%, as shown by Subrahmanyam[13,16], and it certainly reduces the duration of hospitalization.

WHICH HONEY IS THE BEST FOR WOUND TREATMENT?

No laws forbid you to treat the burns of your own daughter when you are on your own in the middle of nowhere. However, if you want to buy honey for wound care from a pharmacy the product must meet pharmaceutical standards. According to the law of most western countries one has to make a strict distinction between foods and medicines. So we have to accept that honey cannot be called a medicine. However, in wound care, honey can be registered as a so-called 'medical device'. A pacemaker is for instance a medical device, and so are the instruments used in the operating theatre. Wound dressings to cover open wounds such as Opsite® and Duoderm® are also classified as medical devices. Since July 1999 the Therapeutic Goods Administration (TGA) of Australia has allowed the use of Medihoney® in Australia (but not any honey) as a primary dressing to treat wounds. Australia is therefore the first country in the world that accepts honey as a registered medical device. Medihoney (100% honey) is currently being used clinically in hospitals and by other health-care professionals.

In 2001 two other honey products for which registration has been applied, are also currently being tested in a few hospitals. HoneySoft® (Mediprof, Moerkapelle; The Netherlands) is a combination of a neutral woven carrier of ethylvinylacetate (EVC) and pure honey within a patented plaster[12]. Mesitin® (Triticum bv, Maastricht, The Netherlands), the second honey product, is quite different because it is a sterile mixture of honey and a number of non-honey substances (e.g. low allergic lanolin, sunflower oil, zinc oxide). Mesitin has many things in common with Desitin, a product registered by Carl Klinke (Hamburg, Germany) that had a very good reputation in the thirties (1935). Desitin ointment was used for the treatment of burns and other wounds. Both Lücke and Buchheister reported excellent results with Desitin[18,19]. Carl Klinke's factory closed during World War II, and Desitin ceased production.

It should be noted here that Mesitin is not simply a copy of Desitin. For instance the antibacterial activity of honey is now well defined, which was not possible in 1935. Some additional substances have been added to improve the ointment, and the product is now patent pending (see www.triticum.nl).

The rediscovery of honey in this millennium and its registration as a medical device will turn a 5000 year old folk remedy into an clinically accepted wound dressing of today.

REFERENCES

1. MARSDEN, A K; MOFFAT, C; SCOTT, R (1995) *First aid manual. Authorized manual of St John Ambulance, St Andrew's Ambulance Association and the British Red Cross.* Dorling Kindersley; London, UK; pp 103–112 (revised 6th edition).

2. LAWRENCE, J C (1986) *Burncare*. Presented at a British Burn Association teaching symposium, Hull, UK (unpublished).

3. ARTURSON, G (1991) Management of burns. *Proceedings of the 1st European conference on advances in wound management, 4–6 September 1991*; pp 135–141.

4. RIJN, O VAN (1991) *Burn injuries among young children. Incidence, aethiology and determinants of behavioral risk factors*. Thesis, University of Maastricht, the Netherlands.

5. DROUET, N (1983) L'utilisation du sucre et du miel dans le traitement des plaies infectées. *Press Med* 12: 2355–2356.

6. KEITH, J F; KNODEL, L C (1988) Sugar in wound healing. *Drug Intell Clin Pharm*. 22: 409–411.

7. WHITE, J W; SUBERS, M H; SHEPARTZ, A I (1963) The identification of inhibine, the antibacterial factor in honey, as hydrogen peroxide and its origin in a honey glucoseoxidase system. *Biochem Biophys Acta* 73: 57–70.

8. KERKVLIET, J D (1996) Screening method for the determination of peroxide accumulation in honey and relation with HMF content. *Journal of Apicultural Research* 35: 110–117.

9. WHITE, J W; SUBERS, M H (1963) Studies on honey inhibine. 2. A chemical assay. *Journal of Apicultural Research* 2: 93–100.

10. POSTMES, T J; BOSCH, M M C; DUTRIEUX, R; BAARE, J VAN; HOEKSTRA, M J (1997) Speeding up the healing of burns with honey. In Mizrahi, A; Lensky, Y (eds) *Bee products: properties, applications and apitherapy*. Plenum Press; New York, USA; pp 57–63.

11. HOEKSTRA, M J; HUPKENS, P; DUTRIEUX, R P; BOSCH, M M C; KREIS, R W (1993) A comparative burn wound model in the New Yorkshire Pig for the histopathological evaluation of local therapeutic regimens: silver sulfadiazine cream as standard. *Britsih Journal of Plastic Surgery* 46: 585–589.

12. HOEKSTRA, H; PONT, J S DU; DUTRIEUX, R P (1999) Honey-Soft een bij-zonder verband met artsen van het LCPL. *Gevangen in het neurale net. Jaarverslag 1999 Leids cytologisch Pathologisch Laboratorium*; Leiden, the Netherlands; p 40.

13. SUBRAHMANYAM, M (1991) Topical application of honey in treatment of burns. *Br J Surg* 78: 479.

14. LOCKHART, S P; RUSHWORTH, A; AZMY, A A F et al. (1984) Topical silver sulphadiazine: side effects and urinary excretion. *Burns* 10: 9–12.

15. CHOBAN, P S; MARSHALL, W J (1987) Leukopenia secondary to silver sulfadiazine. Frequency, characteristics, and clinical consequences. *Am Surg* 53: 515–517.

16. SUBRAHMANYAM, M (1996) Honey dressing for burns – an appraisal. *Ann Burns and Fire Dis* 9: 33–35.

17. EFEM, S E E (1988) Clinical observations on the wound healing properties of honey. *British Journal of Surgery* 75: 679–681.

18. BUCHHEISTER, H (1935) Erfahrungen mit Honig und Lebertran in der Wundbehandlung. *Münchener Med Wochenschrift* (40): 1612–1613.

19. LÜCKE, H (1935) Wundbehandlung mit Honig und Lebertran. *Deutsche Med Wochenschrift* 61: 1638–1640.

THEO POSTMES
Biomedical Research Foundation, Maastricht, The Netherlands

Appendix: Botulism and honey

CLIFF VAN EATON

Some paediatricians have recommended that honey should not be fed to infants less than one year old because of the possibility that *Clostridium botulinum* spores may be present in the honey[6]. *C. botulinum* is the causative organism of botulism. Spores of the organism do not germinate in the acidic adult digestive system, but may germinate in the gut of young infants because they do not have a well-developed intestinal flora. Ninety-four per cent of infants hospitalized with botulism are between the ages of two weeks and six months[1].

Cases of infant botulism, and all botulism disease, are rare. Since 1973, an average of 24 cases of food-borne botulism, three cases of wound botulism, and 71 cases of infant botulism have been reported annually to the US Centres for Disease Control and Prevention[25]. The risk of a child less than one year old contracting infant botulism has been estimated to be about 1 in 12 000[18]. The first cases (2) of food-borne (adult) botulism were recorded in New Zealand in 1985[11]. The cases were not related to honey. A Medline search of 'infant botulism' and 'New Zealand" for the past 20 years did not reveal any records.

Spores of *C. botulinum* were first identified in several samples of honey in California in 1976[15]. Midura *et al.*[20] found spores of the organism in 10% of retail samples. Using the same method described by Midura *et al.*, 107 samples of honey sold in Italy were examined, but no spores of the organism were found[3]. Huhtanen, *et al.*,[15] using the same method found no spores in 80 samples of honey sold in the USA, but using another method, found spores in 6 samples. Surveys in Italy[23], France[8], Norway[14], and two large surveys in Germany[12,13] also did not find spores of *C. botulinum* in honey samples. A further study of 56 samples of honey sold in Germany found spores of *C. perfringens* (7 samples), and *C. sphenoides* and *C. butyricum* (1 each), but no *C. botulinum* spores[5]. In Argentina, following a report from Japan of *C. botulinum* spores in Argentinian honey, a survey was conducted that found spores in 1.1% of 177 samples, 68 of which were from commercial origin[9].

In the original California study[2], *C. botulinum* spores, but no pre-formed toxin, were identified in 6 honey samples that had been previously fed to 3 patients with infant botulism. Food exposure studies also showed that 29% (12/41) of hospitalized patients had been fed honey. However, the study concluded that the distribution of spores was ubiquitous (soil, air, etc.), and only recommended that honey not be fed to infants because it was an avoidable source of *C. botulinum* spores.

Subsequent research has determined that *C. botulinum* spores are not only present in the soil, but are more widespread in corn syrup than in honey (20% compared to 2%), and occur in infant foods, cereals, milk, and fruit and vegetable preparations[16]. By the mid-1980s, honey had not been proven to cause infant botulism, but was still being suggested as a risk factor associated with the condition[18].

A major epidemiological study of infant botulism in the US State of Pennsylvania identified breast-feeding as the major link with the disease. Honey was determined to not be a causative factor, with environmental conditions (soil, dust) implicated instead as the major and unavoidable source of spores[19].

Spika, *et al.*[26] defined risk factors for infant botulism in 68 cases in the US. Breast feeding posed the greatest risk (odds ratio = 2.9), followed by decreased frequency of bowel movement (odds ratio = 5.2) and honey consumption (odds ratio = 9.8), although only 16% of the patients had eaten honey. Risk factors also changed depending on the age of the infant, with living in a rural area being the only significant risk factor for infants under 2 months of age (odds ratio = 6.4). With infants over 2 months the most important factors were reduced bowel movement (odds ratio = 2.9), breast feeding (odds ratio = 3.8) and ingestion of corn syrup (odds ratio = 5.2). The report concluded that food exposures account for the minority of cases of infant botulism, with pre-existing host factors such as intestinal flora and frequency of bowel movements being the most important risk factors.

Honey continues to periodically be reported in the literature as a potential risk factor associated with infant botulism. For instance, a Japanese paper[21] reported 13 cases of infant botulism with only one with no previous history of honey ingestion, but also suggested that other cases in which honey was not a factor may not have been diagnosed.

The first record of a confirmed case of infant botulism caused from honey in Europe is reported by Fenicia *et al.*[10]. In this case, spores of the same strain of *C. botulinum* were isolated from the patient and from a jar of home-produced honey that had been used to sweeten the pacifier of the baby. The assumption made by the authors is that the honey was the source of the infection. Another report from Denmark[4] linked the same strain of *C. botulinum* with the patient and a brand of honey (but not the specific container) that had been fed to the baby.

Fives cases of infant botulism were recorded in a one-year period in a province of Argentina[22]. *C. botulinum* spores were not detected in samples of honey that had been fed to two of the patients prior to onset of the disease.

There does not appear to have been any detailed survey of New Zealand for the presence of *C. botulinum* spores, although export consignments are sometimes analysed for the presence of spores by analytical labs. No countries appear to have government requirements for the testing of honey imports for *C. botulinum* spores[24].

Because of the high sugar content of honey (about 82%), if the product is stored properly, no micro-organisms, including *C. botulinum*, are able to grow in the product, and toxins will not be produced. The presence of *C. botulinum* spores in honey is not the result of poor processing or bottling, and the spores, if they are present, cannot be eliminated under normal conditions unless ultrafiltration is used. Heating food products to 80°C for several minutes will destroy *C. botulinum* and its toxin, but the spores persist up to 130°C[17]. Heating honey to this level would significantly alter the product's essential composition and impair its quality, and would lead to hydroxymethylfurfural (HMF) levels above the maximum allowed under Codex Alimentarius[7].

References

1. ARNON, S (1986) Infant botulism: anticipating the second decade. *Journal of Infectious Diseases* 154(2): 201–206.
2. ARNON, S and 5 others (1979) Honey and other environmental risk factors for infant botulism. *Journal of Pediatrics* 94(2): 331–336.
3. AUREIL, P; FERRINI, A; NEGRI, S (1983) *Clostridium botulinum* spores in honey. *Rivista Della Soc. Ital. Sci. dell'aliment* 12: 457–460.
4. BALSLEV, T and 3 others (1997) Infant botulism; the first culture-confirmed Danish case. *Neuropediatrics* 28(5): 287–8.
5. BENTLER, W; FRESE, E (1981) Mikrobielle Bescaffenheit und Rukstandsuntersuchungen von Bienenhonig. *Archiv Lebensmittelhygiene* 32(4): 130–135.
6. BROWN, L (1979) Infant botulism and the honey connection. *Journal of Pediatrics* 94(2): 337–338.
7. CODEX ALIMENTARIUS COMMISSION (1994) *Honey*. Food and Agriculture Organisation of the United Nations and the World Health Organisation; Rome, Italy (2nd edition).
8. COLIN, M and 3 others (1986) La qualite des miels du commerce. *Cah. Nut. Diet* 21(3): 219–222.
9. DE CENTORBI, O and 4 others (1997) Detection of *Clostridium botulinum* spores in honey. *Rev Argent Microbiol* 29(3): 147–51.
10. FENICIA, L and 3 others (1993) A case of infant botulism associated with honey feeding in Italy. *European Journal of Epidemiology* 9(6): 671–3.
11. FLACK, L (1985) Botulism in New Zealand. *New Zealand Medical Journal* 98: 892–3.
12. FLEMMIG, R; STOJANOWIC, V (1980) Untersuchungen von Bienenhonig auf *Clostridium botulinum* Sporen. *Arch. Lebensmittelhygiene* 31(5): 179–180.
13. HARTGEN, H (1980) Untersuchungen von Honigproben auf Botulinus-toxin. *Arch. Lebensmittelhygiene* 31(5): 177–178.
14. HETLAND, A (1986) *Clostridium botulinum* sprer i norskproduserd honning? *Norsk. Vet. Artidsskr.* 98(10): 725–727.
15. HUHTANEN, C; KNOX, D; SHIMANUKI, H (1981) Incidence and origin of *Clostridium botulinum* spores in honey. *Journal of Food Protection* 44(11): 812–814.
16. KAUTTER, D; LILLY, T; SOLOMON, H; LYNT, R (1982) *Clostridium botulinum* spores in infant foods: a survey. *Journal of Food Protection* 45(11): 1028–1029.
17. KRELL, R (1996) *Value-added products from beekeeping*. Food and Agriculture Organisation of the United Nations, FAO Agricultural Services Bulletin 124; Rome, Italy; p. 51.
18. LAWRENCE, W (1986) Infant botulism and its relationship to honey: a review. *American Bee Journal* 126: 484–486.
19. LONG, S (1985) Epidemiologic study of infant botulism in Pennsylvania: report of the infant botulism study group. *Pediatrics* 75(5): 928–934.
20. MIDURA, T and 3 others (1979) Isolation of *Clostridium botulinum* from honey. *Journal of Clinical Microbiology* 9(2): 282–283.
21. MORIKAWA, Y and 4 others (1994) A case report of infant botulism without a history of honey ingestion. *Kansenshogaku Zasshi* 68(2): 259–62.
22. PUIG DE CENTORBI, O and 4 others (1998) Infant botulism during a one year period in San Luis, Argentina. *Zentralbl Bakteriol* 287(1–2): 61–6.
23. QUAGLIO, P; MESSI, P; FABIO, A (1988) An investigation about the presence of bacteria of the genus *Clostridium* in honey samples *L'Igiene Moderna* 15(3): 486–496.
24. REID, M (1999) Manager, New Zealand Honey Export Certification. (Personal communication).
25. SHAPIRO, R; HATHEWAY, C; SWERDLOW, D (1998) Botulism in the United States: a clinical and epidemiologic review. *Ann Intern Med* 129(3): 221–8.

CLIFF VAN EATON

Apiculture Scientist, Horticulture Research NZ Ltd, Hamilton, New Zealand

www.ingramcontent.com/pod-product-compliance
Lightning Source LLC
Chambersburg PA
CBHW080554170426
43195CB00016B/2793